Thousands of books have been written about weight loss, so why read Cracking the Weight Loss Code? Well since diets are clearly not the most effective approach to this challenge, finding a holistic, mind-body approach is what many people are seeking in order to tackle the problem of being overweight.

Stina brings an integrative approach as a nutritionist, healing practitioner as well as her direct personal experience to this step by step guide to discovering what often sabotages those who try with great effort to lose the pounds they desire.

Unconscious factors that often stem from unsuccessful prior attempts as well as self-defeating thoughts, feelings and belief can undercut even the most motivated of individuals who find themselves on this path and this book offers powerful insight and guidance for how to navigate and overcome many of these invisible saboteurs.

Craig Weiner, D.C., Director of the EFT Tapping Training Institute

"Delightfully astounded! I am amazed at the wonderful straightforward approach to this challenge that over 80% of North Americans struggle with. A seemingly insurmountable problem becomes a stepping stone toward personal freedom and peace with these simple, beautifully orchestrated options for release.

The skillful methods described by Nutrition/ Transformation Coach Stina Pope are timely, relevant for any issue, and accessible to all; at any time of day and any season of life. I only wonder what possibilities this will open for you. Of what would you like to be free? What is making the next step toward that option hard for you? Are you ready and willing to let it go? What might it feel like once you're on the other side of this issue?"

Marcia J Howton, MD, ASA Board Certified Anesthesiologist; IBPM Board Certified Pain Management; Co-author Andrew Weil Integrative Medicine Series; Integrative Pain Management, Chapter on Mindfulness in Medicine; Instructor on Mindfulness Based Stress Reduction and Mindfulness Based Cognitive Therapy; Trained Trauma Resolution Specialist for Holographic Memory Resolution, Feeding Your Demons, Neurolinguistic Programming, and Medical Hypnosis.

Cracking the Weight Loss Code

Tools That Work

by

Stina Pope

ISBN: 979-8-9862356-1-5   eISBN: 979-8-9862356-0-8

Cover Design: Arjan van Woensel

Editor: Jeremy Anderson

An Important Note to Readers

The author of this book does not dispense medical advice or prescribe the use of any technique as a form of treatment for physical, emotional, or medical problems without the advice of a physician or mental health professional, either directly or indirectly. As with all new food, fitness, and mental health regimens, any changes you make in this arena should be followed only after first consulting with a doctor to make sure it is appropriate for your individual circumstances.

Nutritional and emotional needs vary from person to person, depending on age, sex, health status, medication requirements and total diet.

The intent of the author is only to offer educational information of a general nature to help you in your quest for physical, emotional and spiritual well-being. In the event you use any of the information in this book for yourself, the author and the publisher assume no responsibility for your actions.

Preface

Why another book on releasing weight? After the birth of my second child, a divorce, and one life-upheaval after another for years on end, I was not surprised to find the addition of more pounds each year. I tried one thing after another, most did not work, some worked backwards, and I despaired. When I was introduced to EFT-Tapping, I began to have hope. It worked. I got a masters degree in holistic health and began to understand why it worked. When I was introduced to the technique of BSFF™, I knew I had found an additional and important game-changer. With my extensive background in nutrition and body-mind techniques, I want to share these tools that work.

This is a book about releasing excess weight that has gathered in and on one's body. And it does that by teaching a system that will enable you to let go of anything that weighs you down. The tools you will learn in this book have the potential to release all kinds of things which are not helpful to you, bringing you into alignment and coherence. If you find these tools helpful, I am blessed.

I want to give thanks, first to Brad Yates. At a tapping seminar in Seattle, he worked with me as I fumbled around saying I wanted to write a book. Well, Brad, here it is.

One of Brad's multitudinous YouTube tapping videos introduced me to the name of Larry Nims, who created the Be Set Free Fast™ (BSFF) Program. That introduction leads me to say thank you so much to both Larry Nims, PhD, and Alfred Heath, MA, for their careful guidance and the permission to use the BSFF™ work here. Please note: This book is not aimed at training you to be a practitioner/provider of BSFF™, but you will learn how to use it for yourself.

And then there is the research of Dr. Peta Stapleton showing that EFT meridian tapping made as much of a difference in initial weight loss as CBT (Cognitive Behavioral Therapy), the current gold standard for weight loss. That is significant enough, but then she showed that EFT clearly outperformed CBT over time in weight loss maintenance. Her research, concepts and support were instrumental in the creation of this book. Thank you so much, Peta.

(Please see the **Resources** at the end for more information on each of these people and their work.)

Finally, thanks to Sue, my incredible partner and spouse, who has believed in me and kept me going for so many years.

Cracking the Code

Tools to Release Weight

Introduction

You will find a novel approach to releasing weight here, one that is interested in bringing you back to who you are as a healthy human being, on a very fundamental level. You will learn skills that will bring you into deep alignment with yourself, a coherence that will let you release the things that are not helping you, and will give you a sense of security that you may not even have known was an issue.

When you feel secure, are in alignment, and have coherence, there is deep peace. You will have cracked the code. You may find yourself putting many burdens down.

This book is dense. There is a whole lot of information here, so do not expect to get through it quickly. It is designed to help you go deep and come out in a better place.

Give yourself plenty of time - 6 months is recommended. You want it to be permanent this time. We're talking real transformation.

Read a bit, ponder, write a little in the downloadable journal (see Appendix F, or stinasway.com) or your own journal, then come back and read a little more. Ten minutes a day, maybe every day, maybe twice a week. If you will do it every week, ten minutes is a good time to allot to this work, and it will change your life. Put it in your calendar.

So, welcome! I'm very glad you're here.

Table of Contents

Cracking The Code
Section One
Crack the Emotional Weight Code

WHEN THE WHY IS CLEAR,
THE WAY CAN BECOME CLEAR

Initial Questions

Here are some initial questions to ask yourself:

> Are you calm and stable within yourself?
>
> Do you feel safe in the world, safe to be yourself?
>
> Do you feel you are enough, have enough, are good enough?
>
> Do you have critical self talk?
>
> Do your actions match your intentions?
>
> Do you make the same mistakes even though you told yourself you would not?
>
> Are you often irritated and upset, whether you show it on the outside or not?

How we feel and act in the world indicate underlying problems. False beliefs about ourselves and the world can be factors in holding onto weight. How you answer these questions will help you understand why you eat the way you do and, with the tools provided, release emotional burdens which lead to unproductive eating behavior. We are going to look first at WHY you eat what you eat. Eventually, we will get to WHAT you eat. It turns out that if you deal with the why first, the what is much easier to deal with.

It's not just about the food. When our emotional state is not calm, the body can choose to hold or release weight, no matter what we eat or don't eat. This is why we start with the emotional work, and then go on to the food.

Part 1 - Weight Issues
Basic Assumptions

Dealing with weight is typically a difficult and long-standing issue. Here are the basic assumptions we will be using.

- The saying "mind over matter" is true. If you don't deal with the mind issues that affect the weight you are carrying, you can power through losing some, but it will come back.

  - *You will learn how to heal the mind issues (crack the code) with powerful tools.*

- If you knew how to release weight and keep it off, you would have done so. You are not stupid, you just didn't have enough of the right tools, and it does take a multi-pronged approach.

  - *With the tools you learn here, you will understand what you need to do to release weight permanently.*

- There is no one food program that fits everyone.

  - *You will learn how to discern what works for you.*

- Insulin makes you gain weight. Each time you have an insulin "hit", you increase the potential to store fat.

  - *You will learn how to increase your resistance to gaining weight.*

- Inflammation is both a good thing and a very bad thing.

    - *You will learn to tell the difference, and how to release the bad.*

- Exercise makes you healthier. It does not help you lose weight.

    - *Yes, movement is good, but do it so you get healthier and feel better. You'll get ideas about the best movement for you.*

- If you don't clean out the pipes, you'll probably get/be sick, that is, you probably won't feel really healthy.

    - *If you don't feel healthy, a very slow and gentle detox is something you probably need.*

- For many of us, some of the extra weight we carry has to do with the need for protection, to keep safe. You cannot let go of what has been protecting you (that is, the extra fat) until you learn how to protect yourself in a different manner.

    - *The first major tool you will learn is Protection/Creating Safety.*

- Our subconscious contains beliefs and commands which guide our behavior in life and in relation to food, many of which are false or sabotaging beliefs and commands.

    - *The second major tool is Be Set Free Fast™, or BSFF™, which clears the sabotaging beliefs so you are free to make conscious* *choices. BSFF™ helps your subconscious work FOR you, in alignment with your wishes, rather than against you. BSFF™ is short for Be Set Free Fast™ - an acronym for **B**ehavioral and **E**motional **S**ymptom **E**limination **T**raining **F**or **R**esolving **E**xcess **E**motions: Fear, **A**nger, **S**adness, **T**rauma; BSFF™ is all about aligning your conscious thought and subconscious mind.*

Dealing with your food will be radically different once a) you know how to protect yourself emotionally, b) you have worked through the subconscious beliefs and know how to release anxiety.

Part 2 - Introduction to the Tools:
Breathe, Journal, Create Safety, Be Set Free Fast™

Breathe

Begin with your breath: breathe in and out deeply three times. Try to breathe out longer than in. Count while you breathe. Try breathing in for 4, out for 6, and then increase the count out as it gets easier.

If you have trouble taking a deep breath in, start with blowing out instead. When you breathe out, your body will automatically relax to be able to pull air back in again. You don't have to force it that way. Nice!

What we know now is that doing those three deep breaths activates the vagus nerve. This automatically reminds the body's nervous system to calm down. Since almost everything to do with releasing weight has an emotional component, knowing how to calm your system is critical.

I will occasionally remind you to breathe, and this three-breath work is what I'm suggesting you do. Any time you feel like something is not quite right or even horribly wrong, start by doing these three breaths. It will help.

Journaling

You should have a journal of some sort to keep notes in. There is a free downloadable journal that goes with this book for your use. See Appendix F or stinasway.com. I want you at the very least to get a binder with some paper and some folders so that you can print things out and keep them in the binder.

Look at the questions I asked you in the Initial Questions. Please write them down in your journal, or pull them up on your online journal. Give yourself plenty of space between each one, and write an initial response. It does not have to be an essay. Just a response, and the date, so you can come back later, look at how the questions hit you now, and answer them again.

Whether or not you want to write down your current weight is somewhat irrelevant, but please do write down your current waist measurement and the date in the back of your journal, or the last page of your binder.

If you know you have sugar issues (including pre-diabetes, Metabolic Syndrome, heart disease, diabetes, or just a serious addiction to sugar) and have not had one recently, ask your doctor for an A1C test to measure your blood sugar levels, or you can go to a lab and get it done. This is the other thing you will put in the back of your journal, with a date.

You may also want to have urinalysis strips so you can check your sugar levels on a regular basis; You can get them online. This is also something that is easy to monitor, and you can keep track of it on the last page as well. The urinalysis numbers are not as accurate as the A1C, but normally you only get an A1C once a year.

Wait a minute, you say. Did I just read "heart disease" in that list? Oh yes, and here's why: heart disease often is caused by "sticky" blood causing clots and closures of arteries and such. What makes the blood sticky? Sugar. So in a manner of speaking, diabetes and heart disease are just two sides of the same coin, whether it has been diagnosed or not.

I'm going to suggest that you set up this program for yourself in your calendar. You know how much emotional time/space you have to take on a life-changing program. This program can be done well in 10 minute chunks - if you stay with it. Some folks have more time than that, more energy, etc. But if not, 10 minutes is still workable, if you will stay with it.

The biggest issue is keeping at it, and your calendar can help you remember to come back. Don't feel ANY guilt if you need to move the next step to the next day, week, or two weeks out.

If you have a major emergency, then move the notification to the next month, to decide when you will get back with the program. It's okay. Just decide that you're going to keep coming back to it. You're worth it.

CREATE SAFETY FOR YOURSELF, AND
YOU CREATE IT FOR THOSE
AROUND YOU

Protection - Creating Safety

When you create safety for yourself, you are also creating it for everyone around you. The protection exercise "Shields Up" involves visualizing a special protective sphere or shield around you. It is customized to be powerful protection against specific threats, and to be comfortable and safe inside.

Often we don't even know that lack of safety or a need for protection is an issue. When talking with a client, she suddenly realized that there was a good reason she could not get rid of the belly fat. As a child, she had been hit repeatedly in the stomach. Her body was doing the best it could for her. Once she realized this, she could emotionally protect herself differently, and then her body could release the physical protection.

DO YOU DO WHAT YOU SAY
YOU ARE GOING TO DO, OR NOT?

BSFF™ - Be Set Free Fast™

When you get your protection shields going, and you feel comfortable reminding yourself to have Shields Up, then you can start doing the BSFF™ process.

The BSFF™ process directly addresses the issues of alignment and coherence. By "alignment" we mean our conscious parts (what we say we are going to do) and subconscious parts (what we actually do) are in agreement - our "inner voices" are working to aid our conscious goals.

By "coherence" we mean feeling balanced, connected to our deepest selves, to others, and to life. As you might expect, coherence is much easier to feel if all parts of your mind are acting in harmony and unity. (See heartmath.com for a detailed explanation of coherence and why it is so important.)

When we find ourselves unable to do what we say we are going to do, we are not in alignment and therefore our body-mind lacks coherence. Our subconscious mind is acting in a way that sabotages our conscious goals and intentions. Bringing them into alignment with each other so that there is coherence is what the BSFF™ system does, simply and profoundly.

When we use the BSFF™ system, we find that we are actually able to do what we say we want to do, because we are in alignment.

ALIGNMENT:
BEING IN A POSITION OF AGREEMENT,
A CORRECT ARRANGEMENT OF PARTS

COHERENCE:
FEELING BALANCED, CONNECTED
TO OUR DEEPEST SELVES,
TO OTHERS, TO LIFE

Be Set Free Fast™, or BSFF™, was developed by Larry Nims, PhD and refined by Alfred Heath, MA. This system helps reveal what is true - what we really want - and then shifts the subconscious to be in alignment with the conscious mind. BSFF™ helps your subconscious work FOR you, in alignment with your conscious desires, rather than against you.

After doing some preparation, you will learn how to neutralize subconscious beliefs and commands using BSFF™. There are a lot of scripts provided for your use, with guidance on how to use them.

It can look rather overwhelming, but it actually goes quite quickly once you get into it. You will end up with just a few very important issues to work with. These will be the ones you put in your journal to wrestle with over a longer period of time - but there will not likely be too many of these. It's just that these few are critical.

When you feel comfortable adding BSFF™ in to your life is up to you. About 10 minutes at a time is enough to schedule for doing that. There's an initial learning piece of preparation and then the work itself. It's broken up into sections, so doing a section or two is plenty for one day. You can certainly do more if you want, of course!

I want to be honest about the preparation time for BSFF™. The total time for the preparation will normally take more than 10 minutes, unless you already know how to do muscle testing. You can do it in segments. It is not nasty, but it is not the easiest thing to do either.

All I can really say is that it is well worth it. If you will do it, you will have immediate access to the alignment of conscious and subconscious, and the subsequent coherence that leads to deep peace.

These two mental tools have the potential to change your entire life. Yes, the expectation is that you will release weight, but our expectation is that you will also release anxiety, fear, sadness and who knows what else!

ANALYSIS, NOT JUDGMENT

Protection - Creating Safety

In our society, women are usually taught **not** to protect themselves. (Does this tool work for men? Yes, it does.)

This protection exercise is a powerful and elegant way for you to protect yourself. The customized visualization of a special protective 'shield' or sphere is amazingly useful, powerful, and protective. You will set it up to be powerful protection against specific threats, and to be comfortable and safe inside. We can and should use 'Shields Up' in almost all situations.

> Imagine, just as you sit there, that you have a sphere around you, a sphere of energy. Is the air clean in your sphere? If not, grab a golden feather duster from the ground and clean it out until it feels nice and sparkly in there. (This is a great exercise to teach children.)

> Look at how big your sphere is, and make it big, as big as the room, and how does that feel? Now bring it in so it is very close around you, and how does that feel?

> Push it out again, and then slowly bring it back in until you feel the "click" of the set point, which should still leave you room to dance. (Think about the DaVinci human in the circle. Your sphere should be at least that big, if not bigger.)

Now look at the surface of your sphere; How thick is it? Make it thicker. In this environment, everything can be made transparent and nothing has weight.

Up in the corner of the room, you see there is a tiny TV, and up pops the face of someone who has said something that hurt you. It doesn't matter whether it was intentional or not, just whether it hurt.

As you are looking, that person turns into a cartoon, and the hurtful words that were said come out in a word bubble. Study those words for a minute, and watch the hurtful words turn into hurtful things, physical things. What are those things?

Is the outside of your sphere strong enough and *calibrated to withstand those specific things*? If not, reinforce it. You can make layers, until you are ready, and then you let those things come at your sphere. What happens? Do any of them stick? Do any of them get in??

Rewind the action until, when you give the OK and those things come at you, the hurtful things simply slide off, with no impact. They should be like a mosquito on the rhinoceros hide, irrelevant.

We are pretending here: we pretend that the hurtful words turn into hurtful things, like swords, and we pretend that we have steel on the outside of our spheres, which makes the swords irrelevant.

The interesting thing is that the more attentive we are to exactly what those hurtful things are, and attentive to how exactly, in the physical realm, we would choose to protect ourselves against them, the better this all works. We want to calibrate the shielding to deal just with the hurtful things, and nothing more.

Now look at the face on the screen again. Is this person going to get disgusted and walk off, or will they up the ante? If they walk off, then change the channel to the next person and what they said, and do the process again.

If they are likely to up the ante, pause the action and think about how much more protection you are going to need, and install it.

When you are totally ready, let them throw whatever. Take a good look at your protection, install more as needed, until even these serious attacks become irrelevant.

Usually it takes a while to figure out exactly what kind of and how much protection we need. Just keep playing around with this, and ponder what you want to have ready for when something totally appalling happens.

The outside of your protective shield should usually be something that is clearly identified as strong and boring, like gunmetal gray. You want a bully to look at it and quickly say, "never mind."

The inside of your sphere is totally different. This is your happy place. Don't worry about physical reality here, you can have streams, trees, silk scarves and beautiful artwork, whatever makes you happy.

And this is totally your space! No other person ever gets in here. When you want to be intimate with someone, you have already learned that you can bring the edge of the sphere right up next to your physical skin, and that's just fine - but only you are allowed inside your emotional skin.

A shoe analogy shows how protection should be automatic and fit the situation. It takes me a good while to find shoes that work for me, but once I find them, I am ready for any situation.

I make an **analysis of what I need**, which is based on the weather, where I am walking, the social setting etc., **not a judgment** when thinking about which shoes I will put on. I say, "oh, it's raining, I need rain boots," I don't say "bad rain." The same thing goes for putting up our protective shields. Make an analysis, not a judgment! Customize the shield to the situation.

Why would I not wear shoes?

Why would I not protect myself?

Many of us have been taught that if we protect ourselves emotionally, we will not be loved. It is a lie, a big and very nasty lie. The truth is, if we protect ourselves, we not only create safety for ourselves, but for those around us. Remember the airline mantra: Put your own mask on first, so you can help someone else, and so you don't end up needing to be helped.

If you are not protected, you have three options: you get hit—you are the victim; you hit others first—you are the bully; or you run—your options are controlled by what threatens you.

When you protect yourself with Shields Up, you do not need to be the victim, you do not need to be the bully, and you do not need to run. You may choose to leave the situation, but that is different than having to run away so you don't get hurt.

Analysis is the name of the game. When you have at least some level of protection up, you can get quite curious about how you get hit, by whom, and in what situations. Just as you choose particular garments for dealing with a blizzard, you also want to choose particular layers for your protection when dealing with certain people and situations. Guess what? It won't work beautifully all the time. However, you will get more adept, and life gets a lot nicer.

When a part of the protection doesn't work, just retreat (the bathroom is a great place for this), analyze what is not working, and put up enormous amounts of new protection, and walk back out again, being curious about what they will try next.

Analyze the next set of people you will be dealing with, and what layers you may need, and just go ahead and install the layers. So every time you are dealing with others, via text, phone, email, or even snail mail, put your shields up. This includes the people who love us the most, because it's not about intention. They don't intend to hurt us, and sometimes they do. Shields Up!

And what does this have to do with weight? Simply this: If you don't feel protected, your body will do the job for you. Once you start protecting yourself emotionally as a normal everyday thing, then you are in a position to talk to the body and tell it to let go; that it's OK to let it go; that you don't need the weight to protect you any more.

You say thank you to your body for keeping you alive during some hard times. And you may want to go back to some of those hard times, and teach your earlier self how to put up protection. But that comes after you feel comfortable with using it in your everyday life now.

For some of you, this will not be new. That's fine, just read through the material, do the exercise, put a reminder into your calendar to do "Shields Up" for the next 21 days so it becomes an easy habit: something you automatically do, like putting your shoes on before going outside.

For others, this may be new territory. In either case, feel very free to play around with it, trying on new and different types of protection/shielding, remembering times when you got hit (ouch) as a way of learning what you need to put up for protection now.

Read through the directions until you have internalized them. This will usually take 10 min, a few minutes to read the section, and a few minutes to decide how it should look for today.

26

WHEN INTENTIONS AND BELIEFS
ARE ALIGNED,
WE FEEL COHERENCE, DEEP PEACE

Be Set Free Fast™
Tutorial

BSFF™ is all about aligning the intentions of your conscious thought with the beliefs of the subconscious. When intentions and beliefs are in alignment, the conscious and subconscious work together, and our entire system is balanced and in coherence.

If alignment is similar to even breathing - something you need for calm but can notice directly and even control directly in short bursts - coherence is like an even heart rate. Having good coherence you just feel better; a sense of deep peace and happiness. Lacking coherence you might feel vaguely crummy and be unable to pin down why. If you're not feeling peace, here's a simple way to get there.

Have you ever realized that you say you are going to do something, and then just don't get around to doing it—or—you say you are not going to do something anymore, and there you are, doing it again? When that happens, the subconscious is overriding the conscious mind, and there is not alignment.

The subconscious is much more powerful than the conscious mind, and it is actively trying to protect us. There's just one problem: The subconscious is operating on beliefs that often come from childhood events, beliefs that the conscious mind may have discarded.

Noticing these inconsistencies of alignment or false beliefs are critical to this process. For example, you say you are not going to eat sweets, and then realize you have done so without even really registering that you were doing something inconsistent with what you just said.

Let's start with some BSFF™ definitions (you'll find them again later in the text and in Appendix E):

- A **problem** is a self-limiting and often upsetting personal experience (thought, emotion, or sensation), condition (physical symptom) or behavior (action or inaction) that has subconscious emotional roots (unresolved emotions from the past) combined with a controlling subconscious belief, creating a "program." *Problems are noticed at the conscious level.*

- A **program** is caused by a past upsetting emotional life experience, the feelings (emotional roots) and thoughts (belief) about which take up lodging in our subconscious mind and are automatically triggered —like a computer program —as a learned response to current life situations.

Programs exist at the subconscious level and manifest problems at the conscious level.

- An **issue** in BSFF™ is a group of related problems. *Issues are noticed at the conscious level.*

- A **belief** is something we have decided is true, which is then acted on at the *subconscious* level.

- The **subconscious** is the aspect of the mind that exists and operates outside of our awareness. It is neither good nor bad, but rather is a faithful servant, following our beliefs with action.

- A **treatment** in BSFF™ is this: notice, say a statement about the belief or action, test for truth, use the cue or key word to neutralize, and test again.

Here is an example of what this might look like. **Problem**: I keep drinking too much coffee. **Program**: If I feel low on energy I have to drink another cup to "refuel." **Issue**: I use food and drink to solve most of my immediate emotional concerns. **Belief**: I have to have high energy all day every day. **Subconscious**: Acting on the belief, the subconscious does not allow me to stop drinking coffee, even when I say I want to.

The genius of BSFF™ is that it provides access to those beliefs held in the subconscious. It then relieves the subconscious of continuing to automatically act on them, and allows the subconscious to come into alignment with the desires of the conscious mind.

The Outline of What's Next

Next you will find three sections: the preparation, the BSFF™ tutorial, and an application for using BSFF™ that does not directly deal with weight. Each of these sections is dependent on the previous one, so please do them in order. You can break them up into small bites, and do about 10 minutes at a time, or whatever works for you.

Preparation for BSFF™

There are three pieces of preparation you need to do in order to do the BSFF™ process.

1) Choose your key word
2) Read the Instructions to the Subconscious (see below)
3) Learn how to test for what the subconscious believes.

Follow the directions below for each part of the preparation. When you have completed them, you will be ready to proceed with using BSFF™ to address an issue.

We will start with the issue of dealing with your internal critical parent.

Please be patient. *You will not have to repeat this preparation part.*

1) Choose your key word (originally called the cue or cue word). The word you use for your key word should be short and easy to say. Ideas for key words are: safe, free, now, here, done, avaunt, shazam, fini, hier, and so on. Later on, you can decide to change your key word, just go back to the first paragraph of the Instructions to the Subconscious, and inform the subconscious that it should now recognize this new word. For the moment, just choose a word for your key word that is short and easy to say. Write it down in your journal/binder. (Forgetting the key word is your subconscious trying to protect you, so write it down.)

2) Reading the Instructions to the Subconscious is next. This is a little like reading a legal document - which is pretty much what it is. Some of the items in here may not make much sense right now. Don't worry about that; your subconscious will remember them for you. Find yourself a quiet 5 minutes and slowly, carefully read it aloud. Once you have done that, you do not need to do it again, although you certainly can choose to review and read it again later.

These instructions are for you, my subconscious mind. Whenever I use my key word, which is _____ (or any other key word that I may later instruct you to use), you will:

- release all of the emotional roots and belief systems controlling the problem or issue that I have consciously or unconsciously noticed;
- release everything that has caused or could cause me to experience this problem or issue again;
- release all of the problems in my mind, emotions, body and spirit that cause me to have a negative experience in any of my energy systems, or to be limited in any way;
- release all issues or problems from every contributing person (past, present, still alive or not), event, situation, or circumstance in my life;
- release any and all hidden beliefs, experiences, emotions, affects or other information which contributed to setting up or maintaining this problem/issue in my experience or which could hinder complete resolution of everything needing treatment; and
- release all of the accumulated mental, emotional, physical and spiritual traumatic stresses that I have ever experienced as a result of this problem or issue during my entire existence;

From this moment on, whenever I use my key word to treat an issue or problem, you will allow all of the critical, protective, and maintenance functions and faculties of my whole being to allow treatment to be optimally thorough, efficient, and effective.

Subconscious, you will also allow these faculties and functions to accept and integrate all treatment benefits, and to adapt, upgrade and integrate all structures, functions, and processes of my whole being accordingly.

During the Closing Sequence:

- when I think or say "All Trauma," and use my key word, you will release any remaining traumatic stress affect from any and all problems that I just treated;

- when I think or say "All Stoppers," and use my key word, you will treat all of the stoppers, including any other problems not on the stoppers list that may act like stoppers;

- when I think or say "Forgive everyone and everything," and use my key word, you will release all of the unforgiveness that I ever experienced toward everyone and everything that I consciously or unconsciously held responsible for one or more of the problems I have just treated;

- when I think or say "Forgive myself for any anger and unforgiveness towards myself," and use my key word, you will eliminate all anger, judgment, criticism, unforgiveness and any related problems that I have directed toward myself for every problem that I treated during my treatment session.

In addition, if I have not completed any of the Closing Sequence steps in any previous treatment sessions, then you will include them as I do each step of the Closing Sequence in my current session.

Also, whenever I am guiding someone in using the BSFF™ self-treatment methodology, you will treat in me any similar problems and issues that the other person is treating—problems that I may also have, and all problems in me that will or could distract me for alertly and skillfully guiding others through their treatment process.
Now say your key word.

> This concludes the instructions to your subconscious mind. Your use of the key word at the end confirms your intention for your subconscious to do all future treatments as instructed. It will always do this for you from now on.

3) The third preparation piece is learning to test for the subconscious belief using your own body wisdom. It is also an effective means of identifying programs. There are several ways to do the testing. You can use muscle testing, a pendulum, the "Quick Y/N" or the Subjective Units of Distress Scale (SUD scale).

Muscle Testing: We will start with muscle testing. Once you learn this skill, you can use it in all sorts of places. Muscle testing is a way to access your own body wisdom. Read through the instructions for doing muscle testing, and see if you can do it. **If not, don't fret, there are other ways.** Try pretending you are a child learning this. Let it be simple, and if it doesn't work right now, just go on to one of the other methods. You can come back to this some time later and try again if you want.

- Please stand up, wiggle your body a little to loosen up, and then say out loud, "My name is ___ " and feel your body move itself forward very subtly. Then you will use someone else's name, and feel your body move itself backward very subtly. If your name is Michael, you would say, "My name is Michael" and feel the forward movement, and then say something like, "My name is Joan" and feel the backward movement. Again, these movements are subtle.

- Shake yourself out a little, and try it again. If you are feeling even just a little bit of that movement, that's enough. What we are doing here is allowing you to register that you can indeed access that body wisdom, which is your access to the subconscious. Practice it a few more times.

- Now, assuming you have felt that subtle movement, sit down, put one hand on your leg where it falls easily, and lift up your forefinger. (If you haven't felt any movement, go on to the next paragraph.) Say the same sentence you used before: My name is _____. Using your other hand, push down on the forefinger. Because you are telling the truth, it should stay strong. Now use

35

the other person's name, and when you push down on the forefinger, it should be weak, because the body recognizes it as false. If your finger gets tired, shake your hand out, go get a glass of water, and come back to this. Muscle testing is a practice - the more you play with it, the more comfortable you will become using it.

- There are several different kinds of muscle testing, some using thumb and finger, some two fingers, and so on. Any of them will do, as long as you are comfortable with using them to access the body wisdom.

Pendulum: You can also access information from the subconscious letting the subconscious/body speak to you through the movement of a pendulum. You will want to test for the Y/N similarly by using your name, saying "My name is __" and then another name that is not yours, or something very simple that is true, like "I'm wearing X color socks." Then use a false statement, "I'm wearing Y color socks." It is important to maintain a curious and disinterested attitude.

If you have not used a pendulum previously and are interested in using this method, full instructions for using one are provided in Appendix C.

Quick Y/N: You can also simply allow yourself to answer the statements below with a quick yes or no. The answer of Y/N needs to be very quick, so your conscious mind doesn't have time to filter what it thinks the appropriate answer is.

You may want to start practicing this with having a friend asking you some questions that they have prepared. They should push you to answer very quickly, preferably questions that ask for yes/no answers. You want to get used to this kind of "answering without thinking" in this context.

SUD Scale: Another way to access the subconscious is using the SUD (Subjective Unit of Discomfort) scale. This is a 0-10 scale. You may have seen something like this in your doctor's office done with both words and faces that can go from no pain (0) to great pain (10). At the beginning of working with the issue of dealing with your critical parent voice, I will ask you to rate 0-10, how intense is the voice of internal critical parent? 0=not intense at all, 10=extremely intense. After doing the exercise, I will ask you what your new number is.

- Please note! There's **no** shame here if you don't get the muscle testing. It was years until someone taught me the Sway Test (which is what I suggest starting with above) that I could suddenly do it. There are a variety of ways to do muscle testing, I think the Sway Test is the easiest.

- If you can do the Sway test but not the finger bit, then just put your paper or laptop on the kitchen counter and stand and sway. And if using a pendulum, the quick Y/N or 0-10 works for you, that's fine. All you need is access to the subconscious, however you get it.

Next Steps

Now that you have completed all of the preparations, you will be rather amazed at how simple the next steps are. (Well, I was.)

Please note! If you are having trouble making sense of any part of this, I highly encourage you to go look at the introduction work you can find at https:// www.bsfftraining.org/a-beginner's-bsff-quickstart. It really makes a big difference watching Dr. Larry Nims do a session. He's the one who created BSFF™, and his work is masterful.

Again, a "treatment" in BSFF™ is simply this:

- *notice the issue,*
- *say a statement* that highlights the belief or action connected to a problem within that issue,
- *test* whether the subconscious' response is a **problem** - that is, if it is out of alignment with what you want consciously,
- if the result highlights a problem, *use your key word* to neutralize it, and
- *test again.*

If the test shows that the problem is still present, there is a Fail-Safe Procedure to address it more directly and deeply (discussed below).

When you see the word "test" this means doing muscle testing, using a pendulum, the quick Y/N or the SUD Scale. Here's the bottom line: If you have used your key word, you have done a treatment. This will make more sense to you as we go along. Just hang in there.

Flow Chart (see the last page of the book for a diagram of the Flow Chart)

Here's a flow chart of how it works, using the belief of "I'm a bad person" as our example. (If you can, please read down or go to Appendix E and print out the Fail-Safe and Closing pages first so they are ready for you.) I would suggest you put a sticky note here, first just read through the Flow Chart section down through the Closing Sequence below, and then come back here and actually work through it.

Notice the problem, what's the belief?

> - I believe I'm a bad person, but I don't think that's true, but I'm afraid that's true underneath, but I don't want it to be true.

Negative statement

> - Say out loud - "I'm a bad person"

Test Y/N

> - If the answer is N, yay! You're in the **clear**. Go to the positive statement

> - a Y answer is a **problem**, as the subconscious is not in alignment with the desires of the conscious mind

> Use your key word, test again, if Y again, repeat as needed

If still Y, use the Fail-Safe Procedure (see below) until you test N

Positive statement

- Say out loud - "I'm basically a good person" Notice that for this statement the values are reversed: Y is **clear**, and N is a **problem**.

Test Y/N

- If N, subconscious still does not agree, use your key word, test again, if N again, repeat a few times

if still N, use the Fail-Safe Procedure until you test Y

- if Y, you're **clear** and done with this statement set

For this exercise we're only doing these two tests of "I'm a bad person" and "I'm a good person". At the end of any set of tests (whether it's one or fifty or more), do the Closing Sequence (see below).

Remember that which answer - Y or N - is a **problem** and which is **clear** will depend on what question you are asking. When the subconscious testing is returning the answer you consciously want - No to "I'm doomed to fail," Yes to "I'm going to make it," and so on - that's when you're clear to move on. That's when your whole body-mind is in alignment. (See the Flow Chart at the end of the book if you like diagrams!)

Fail-Safe Procedure

Treat each problem separately

- I want to be free of this problem. *Test, key word, test*

- I am willing to be free of this problem. *Test, key word, test*

- I am willing to be free of this problem from now on. *Test, key word, test*

- I give myself permission to be free of this problem from now on. *Test, key word, test*

- It's okay for me to be completely free of this problem from now on. *Test, key word, test*

- I deserve to be free of this problem now and from now on. *Test, key word, test*

- It's safe for me to be free of this problem now and from now on. *Test, key word, test*

- I am willing to give up all of the benefits of keeping this problem. *Test, key word, test*

- I am willing to receive all of the positive benefits of being free of this problem. *Test, key word, test*

- I will do everything necessary to ensure that I am free, and remain continually free of this problem from now on. *Test, key word, test*

- There are still one or more problems that will make me keep or take back this problem. *Test, key word, test*

- There is still something in me that will make me keep or take back this problem. *Test, key word, test*

- I am still vulnerable to taking this problem back sometime. *Test, key word, test*

If the Fail-Safe Procedure does not resolve the problem after a few attempts, write the problem down and resolve to return to it later. It may require multiple times revisiting the belief to uproot it, or you may wish to seek other approaches to that particular issue.

THE KEY WORD OPENS
THE SUBCONSCIOUS DOOR,
CLOSE THAT DOOR
WITH THE CLOSING SEQUENCE

The Closing Sequence

A treatment can be using just one statement, or a series of statements, so a BSFF™ treatment can actually take only a minute or two. The question is whether you used your key word. If you have used your key word, you need to use the Closing Sequence.

Normally a treatment will take longer than minutes - but it's helpful to understand that the definition of a *treatment* in BSFF™ is tied to whether you used your key word. If not, you were explaining or getting ready, but not actually doing a treatment.

Each and every time that you use your key word, you want to end your session with the Closing Sequence. Why? Because when we use the key word, we are opening the door to the subconscious. It is important to close that door.

And there can be many other peripheral programs supporting the continued existence or recurrence of the problem you just cleared. In order to be as thorough as possible, you need to clear them too, so that the problem has the least chance of returning. The Closing Sequence offers a comprehensive list to bring closure to the process.

Look carefully at the Closing Sequence. There is a long version to use a few times, and a short version. When you look at the long version of the Closing Statement, you will see a list of "Stoppers."

These are statements that voice our doubts about this process actually working. Giving them voice helps release our doubts. Once you have read through the long version and heard yourself reading the "stoppers" out loud, you can move to the short version. You should be able to memorize the short version very quickly.

The Closing Sequence (long version):

End *every* session (any time you have used your key!) with either version of The Closing Sequence.

1. The Stoppers -

- I am afraid that these treatments won't work for me. *Test, key word, test*

- I am afraid that these treatments won't last. *Test, key word, test*

- I doubt that they will work. *Test, key word, test*

- I doubt that they will last. *Test, key word, test*

- I don't trust myself to do things effectively in these new ways. *Test, key word, test*

- I doubt that I will do things effectively in these new ways. *Test, key word, test*

- I doubt my ability to live out these changes in my life. *Test, key word, test*

- I am vulnerable to taking back one or more of the problems I have treated. *Test, key word, test*

2. I am now treating all my remaining hurt, anger, judgment, criticism, and unforgiveness towards anyone or anything else involved in any of the problems I have treated during this session. *Test, key word, test*

3. I am now treating any leftover trauma or stress still in my being that these problems generated. *Test, key word, test*

4. I am now treating all of my anger, judgment, criticism towards myself for any problem I have treated during this session. *Test, key word, test*

5. I forgive myself for having had any of the problems I have treated during this session. *Test, key word, test*

6. (Optional) Thank you Divine One, I give thanks and praise to you for being with me in all of this

Closing Sequence (the short version): please use the long version a few times first

1. I forgive everyone and everything - key word

2. Now I am treating the Stoppers - key word

3. Now I am treating all leftover stress and trauma - key word

4. Now I am treating for any anger, judgment or criticism toward myself - key word

5. I forgive myself - key word

6. (Optional) God/Divine One, I give thanks and praise to you for being with me in all of this

Practicing With an Issue

When a statement does not neutralize after a few repetitions, use the Fail-Safe Procedure. Then come back and try again. If the statement is still not clear, put it in your journal to come back to work on later.

The issue that we will work with to learn BSFF™ is "I want to be rid of my internal critical parent."

WHEN A CRITICAL PARENT IS PRESENT
YOU ARE NEVER GOOD ENOUGH

Your Internal Critical Parent

Most of us are aware of that "voice" that tells us what we should and should not be doing. On the scale of 0-10 where 0=no problem and 10=high discomfort, what number would you rate the volume or intensity of that voice in your life? Write that number down. Allow yourself to walk through this process, and at the end, ask again what the number is.

Here are a few paragraphs to read about what it means to eliminate your internal critical parent, and then you will see the statements. **You are encouraged to change the statements to make them absolutely pertinent to you, and to add to the list.** You may find it easier to have someone read this aloud to you.

Notice

Noticing is always the beginning point of using BSFF™. When we notice things that are not right somehow, we acknowledge that we are not in alignment. The more we pay attention, the more chance that we have at changing things, and the more we start cracking the code.

Using the tool of BSFF™, we can choose to reprogram ourselves to pay attention, instead of turning away from the pain in our lives. Until we have a way to release the pain, it makes sense to turn away. With these tools, we can follow a different path.

Start by paying attention to your self-talk. Unless you have been making a conscious effort to change your self-talk, you probably still have a critical parent residing in your subconscious mind. If you often use the words *should, ought*, deserve, and *must*, that is a sign that the critical parent is probably in charge.

You can be sure the critical parent is present if you pick on yourself by telling yourself that you are wrong, what you did wrong, complaining about the way you look or behave, pressuring yourself to try harder, or making negative assumptions about the outcome of your efforts.

Living with a critical parent in your head is quite exhausting. The critical parent is demanding, demeaning, and disempowering. No matter what you do, it is never enough and never quite correct. You can never win.

If you listen carefully, you may recognize the voice of your mother, father and/or other authority figures in those messages from your early life. Their critical voices live on until you dismiss them from your subconscious.

If this is one of your issues (and for most of us working on releasing weight, it is, to some extent), learn to pay attention to your self-talk. If you hear that you're criticizing yourself, make an effort to praise yourself instead. That will become easier after you do the following treatment.

I would also suggest that when it comes to weight, we have an external "critical parent" that is social. This "social parent" tells us that we are totally responsible for our being overweight on an individual level. This is simply not true.

Yes, there are things we can do in an individual level, and this book will help you do them. At the same time, there are a wide variety of issues that conspire against us. (See David Berreby below in **Resources**.)

You will find three answers that are helpful in this regard. One is using Shields Up from Creating Safety. Using BSFF™ to release our emotional reaction to this "social parent" is a healthy response, as is using BSFF™ to release our emotional eating trigger reactions. All three of those help us end up happier, being set free.

Here are initial statements for the issue "I want to be rid of the critical parent in my head." *Please feel free to add or substitute statements of your choosing*. I also suggest that you have a copy of the Fail-Safe Procedure and Closing Sequence printed out so that it is ready to use when you work through this set of statements.

You may find it very helpful to

> take a breath,
>
> say the statement,
>
> test, (skip to the end if clear)
>
> use your key word (forcefully if needed),
>
> breathe, and
>
> test again.

Do what feels right to you.

Also, feel free to use a stickie note, flag, ruler or folded paper to keep your place as you move through the statements, especially if you pop over to using the Fail-Safe Procedure, so you don't have any trouble coming back to the original statement.

Just to remind you:

1. Say the statement out loud.

2. Test for whether it is true or not. (If it is clear, move to the next statement.)

3. If there is a problem, use your key word, and test again. Repeat the use of the key word and more testing a few times as needed.

4. If it does not neutralize, pop over to the Fail-Safe Procedure and work the statement through that. Then come back.

5. If it still does not neutralize, put it into your journal and resolve to come back to it.

6. Move on to the next statement.

Before you proceed, what number comes to mind when you think about the "voice" in your head — 0=I don't hear it, 10=I am totally controlled by it. Please write down your number.

Here are your statements for Critical Parent:

- I want to be rid of the critical parent in my head. *Test, key word, test*
- I'm willing to stop picking on myself. *Test, key word, test*
- I deserve to be appreciated. *Test, key word, test*
- I deserve to be acknowledged. *Test, key, test*
- I deserve to be treated like someone I love. *Test, key word, test*
- I am willing to treat myself like someone I love. *Test, key word, test*
- I can accept myself just the way I am. *Test, key word, test*
- I'm willing to accept myself just the way I am. *Test, key word, test*
- I'm a good person and deserve to live without criticism. *Test, key word, test*
- I am enough. *Test, key word, test*
- I have the right be treated well. *Test, key, test*

- It isn't disloyal to my parent to get them out of my head. *Test, key word, test*

- I have the right to set my own standards for myself. *Test, key word, test*

- I can set appropriate standards for myself. *Test, key word, test*

- If I get rid of the critical parent in my head, I will behave better. *Test, key word, test*

- I could do things better if I weren't hearing all of this negative stuff in my head all day. *Test, key word, test*

- The negative talk in my head gives me an excuse for not trying any harder. *Test, key word, test*

- I'm tired of treating myself this way. *Test, key word, test*

- I'm bad because I still don't do what my parents want me to do. *Test, key word, test*

- I can never be a good daughter/son. *Test, key word, test*

- I am a good son/daughter even if I don't do everything my parents want me to do. *Test, key word, test*

- I am a good person even if I don't do everything my parents want me to do. *Test, key word, test*

- I don't need to automatically comply with my parents' expectations of me. *Test, key word, test*

- I don't have to believe what my parents said. *Test, key word, test*

- I don't have to take on their beliefs about themselves. *Test, key word, test*

(You're almost done!)

Here's the Global Statement for this issue:

- I am now treating, in one treatment, all of my need to have a critical parent in my head telling me what to do, and all of the limiting thoughts, beliefs, attitudes, and emotions that would ever make me keep or take back the critical parent in my head. *Test, key word, test*

Take a deep breath. What is the level of your having a critical parent in your head now, 0-10? Go back and look at what you wrote down at the beginning of this section. If this has been a chronic problem, you may have to do the Fail-Safe Procedure several times.

Treat any additional issues that you sense you need to treat during this session, and of course, do the Closing Sequence at the end of each session. For example, you may want to do this section thinking about a critical parent, and then a new session thinking about the "critical social parent."

Also, if you are still having problems with exactly how this is supposed to work, please visit https://www.bsfftraining.org/a-beginner's-bsff-quickstart and watch the videos.

See below for the Closing Sequence and Fail-Safe Procedure. If possible, print them out so you can refer to them easily.

If you have run out of time to complete a section, there is no problem. Just mark it, do the Closing Sequence, and come back to it later.

Fail-Safe Procedure - Treat each problem separately

- I want to be free of this problem. *Test, key, test*
- I am willing to be free of this problem. *Test, key word, test*
- I am willing to be free of this problem from now on. *Test, key word, test*
- I give myself permission to be free of this problem from now on. *Test, key word, test*
- It's okay for me to be completely free of this problem from now on. *Test, key word, test*
- I deserve to be free of this problem now and from now on. *Test, key word, test*
- It's safe for me to be free of this problem now and from now on. *Test, key word, test*
- I am willing to give up all of the benefits of keeping this problem. *Test, key word, test*
- I am willing to receive all of the positive benefits of being free of this problem. *Test, key word, test*
- I will do everything necessary to ensure that I am free, and remain continually free of this problem from now on. *Test, key word, test*

- There are still one or more problems that will make me keep or take back this problem. *Test, key word, test*
- There is still something in me that will make me keep or take back this problem. *Test, key, test*
- I am still vulnerable to taking this problem back sometime. *Test, key word, test*

If the Fail-Safe Procedure does not resolve the problem after a few attempts, write the problem down and resolve to return to it later.

The Closing Sequence (long version)

End **every** session (any time you have used your cue!) with The Closing Sequence (long or short)

1. The Stoppers -

• I am afraid that these treatments won't work for me. *Test, key word, test*

• I am afraid that these treatments won't last. *Test, key word, test*

• I doubt that they will work. *Test, key word, test*

• I doubt that they will last. *Test, key word, test*

• I don't trust myself to do things effectively in these new ways. *Test, key word, test*

• I doubt that I will do things effectively in these new ways. *Test, key word, test*

- I doubt my ability to live out these changes in my life. *Test, key word, test*

- I am vulnerable to taking back one or more of the problems I have treated. *Test, key word, test*

2. I am now treating all my remaining hurt, anger, judgment, criticism, and unforgiveness towards anyone else involved in any of the problems I have treated during this session. *Test, key word, test*

3. I am now treating any leftover trauma or stress still in my being that these problems generated. *Test, key word, test*

4. I am now treating all of my anger, judgment, criticism towards myself for any problem I have treated during this session. *Test, key word, test*

5. I forgive myself for having had any of the problems I have treated during this session. *Test, key word, test*

6. (Optional) Thank you Divine One, I give thanks and praise to you for being with me in all of this

Closing Sequence: (the short version) please read through the long version a few times before using the short version

1. I forgive everyone and everything - key word

2. Now I am treating the Stoppers - key word

55

3. Now I am treating all leftover stress and trauma - key word

4. Now I am treating for any anger, judgment or criticism toward myself - key word

5. I forgive myself - key word

6. (Optional) God/Divine One, I give thanks and praise to you for being with me in all of this

PERMANENT RELEASE OF WEIGHT IS LARGELY THE RESULT OF BEING THOROUGH AT GETTING INTO ALIGNMENT

Now that you have a basic working knowledge of how to do BSFF™ for yourself, I want you to start with writing down your own truths as directed below, then work through the following pages, keeping track of what does not clear immediately. You may want to add them to your list.

Please do not be alarmed by the number of statements in the next section. Often, only one or two statements out of 10-20 do not neutralize quickly (several may not present any problems at all!). The ones that are left are the ones you want to put into your journal so you can come back to them.

As you go through these statements, note the ones that seem particularly important to you, including the ones that used to be true for you—they may have sub-issues lurking. Then come back and work through them until you are confident that you are not holding any of them subconsciously. I encourage you to add test statements for anything that seems appropriate.

Take your time with this. **You are worth the time.** Set aside 10-15 min to work on this a few days a week, and mark it in your calendar.

There are several ways to work with this material. You need to get comfortable with using BSFF™. If the tutorial above was not enough, please refer to the materials on the BSFF™ website at https:/www.bsfftraining.org/. You can also work with a practitioner.

I gave you the issue of "Critical Parent" (not weight) as a tutorial to get used to using BSFF™ because it doesn't take very long, and having the practice will help move you through the weight section much more quickly.

After learning basic BSFF™, start by going through the beginning issues below. Then decide which is easier for you—to deal with the more difficult issues first, knowing that the other ones are easier, or to get easy success with the issues that are not big triggers for you before heading into the big ones.

If you aren't sure, simply work through the sections here in order. If something feels too heavy, move on to another section and come back. Do what feels right for you, but do **something**.

DON'T LOSE WEIGHT, RELEASE IT

BSFF™ for Releasing Weight

Have you noticed that you have gained weight back when you managed to lose it? First, we want to change our language. When you lose your keys, what do you do? You look around and find them. We don't want to lose weight, we want to release it.

This is not just a fancy word change. There are reasons it keeps coming back. If you ignore those reasons, trying harder doing the same things you have done before, you'll have pretty much the same results. Using BSFF™ goes very deep into the subconscious and shifts things there.

Before you go any further (you'll find this in the downloaded journal), write down in the beginning of your online or written journal or binder:

> The date, how you feel right now, and the answers to these questions without thinking too much. Just write, leaving plenty of space between them (take three deep breath now):

- why do you gain weight?
- why do you gain it back?
- how have you lost weight?

Then, write down the answers to these related questions - (if you don't have an answer or the question doesn't apply, just move on to the next)

- what was going on the first time you tried to diet? if you don't remember about the first time, just think back to what you remember about dieting.
- what was going on when you first gained weight?
- what was the response of those around you?

Leave plenty of space, so that you can come back to these answers and add more notes. If you can, give them a number 0-10 (0=no response, 10=hurts a whole lot) that indicates how serious they are or were at the time.

It's fine to say in the past *that* happened, now *this* is going on. For example: after birth of first child, no problem with weight, but after the second, there was. Then think about what else was going on at that time.

After you have worked through some of the rest of this material, you can come back to these statements, read them aloud to yourself, and check again. Have the numbers changed? Write down the new numbers as appropriate, and the date of these new numbers and how you feel.

Issues in BSFF™

For our purposes here:

An **issue** is simply a group of problems.

A **problem** is a set of emotional roots (unresolved emotions from the past) combined with a controlling belief, whether it is true or not.

A **belief** is something we have decided is true, which is then acted on at the subconscious level so it guides our behavior.

People can have vastly different reasons for why they are overweight, in any number of combinations. Some of the usual reasons are that eating is a response to an emotional overload, that the body has been trained to hold weight (which is slightly different from the body not knowing how to *release* weight), the body's metabolism has been reduced, that there is a problem in the endocrine system, that the subconscious feels it is not *safe* to lose weight, and so on.

We now know that weight issues can also be intergenerational, which makes the concept of working to release the subconscious commands even more intriguing and compelling. (See David Berreby in **Resources**.)

Work through the initial list below using BSFF™ to see if any of these issues belong to you. If the initial test answer is clear then simply move on, but if the answer is a problem, use your key word. If the second test is clear, you may want to change the positive statement to a negative one to make very sure.

So, for example, if your key word released the statement "I eat as a response to emotional overload" you would say, "I don't eat as a response to emotional overload." If you have totally cleared this issue, you will know because your muscle testing will deliver an aligned result for both positive and negative questions.

Be ready to jot down new statements as they pop into your mind; Sometimes a specific wording (perhaps related to how you first learned the problematic belief) will

be more meaningful to you than what you read here. Plan on coming back to this self-made list. You may want to mark which issues have caused you the most concern with dates, so you can see your progress as you clear certain parts.

And, as always, finish with the Closing Sequence, no matter how many statements you have worked with.

Initial List

Make a note of what shows up here in your journal

- I eat as a response to an emotional overload. *Test, key word, test*

Go on to the Typical Triggers for Emotional Eating below.

- My body has been trained to hold weight. *Test, key word, test*

Think about working with someone who can help you clear this set of memories.

- My body does not know how to release weight. *Test, key word, test*

Repeat this issue daily for a week using the Fail-Safe Procedure until it lets go. If it doesn't let go after a week, consider working with someone.

- My body's metabolism has been reduced. *Test, key word, test*

Try using the Raising Your Metabolism exercise once every morning until it holds steady

- There is a problem in my endocrine system. *Test, key word, test*

You may want to go to a naturopath and get this tested. Do not assume that it's your thyroid, which can "cover" or "mask" other parts of the system that are the actual problem.

- There is something in my environment that makes me hold weight. *Test, key word, test*

- I have an allergy or major sensitivity that keeps me from releasing weight. *Test, key word, test*

For either of these you may want to go to a chiropractor that does deep allergy testing or go to Sandi Radomski's Allergy Detective work at https://www.rubahomaidi.com

- It is not safe for me to lose weight. *Test, key word, test*

Think about working with someone who can help you clear this set of memories.

- There is some other issue I need to attend to. *Test, key word, test*

Ask yourself to bring this forward for you in dream state, have paper and pen by the bed and write down whatever comes up without judgment.

Wellness List

When we have achieved a state of wellness, we look and feel good. This has very little to do with what the scale says. Plan on coming back to this list as well. Again, you may want to mark dates on which issues have caused you the most concern, so you can see how you have been able to clear certain parts. Remember to breathe.

- I know how to use cues from my physical self to judge how healthy I am. *Test, key word, test*

- I know how to use cues from my mental self to judge how healthy I am. *Test, key word, test*

- I feel buoyant, energetic and agile. *Test, key word, test*

- I have innate wisdom from my body and mind. *Test, key word, test*

- I am strong, fit and well-nourished. *Test, key word, test*

- Movement is a source of joy for me. *Test, key word, test*

- I sit, stand, walk and bend easily. *Test, key word, test*

Alter this for your own movement style if you have a disability that does not permit you to stand or walk.

- Mental clarity and an ability to focus are my norm. *Test, key word, test*

65

- I satisfy my hunger with nourishing, wholesome foods. *Test, key word, test*

It is pretty normal for the Critical Parent to show up right now. You can tell the voice that you are working on the situation, and give them a new job. For example, you can ask the voice to help you identify exact times and places where you have felt these things before. It may have been a small thing, but for most of us, there are times in our lives when some of these things have been true. Redirecting the voice to help us can be a very interesting process. You can also go back and do the Critical Parent script again.

Raising Your Metabolism

Do this exercise in the morning or early afternoon.

Without thinking, answer this question quickly: what percent (between 0-100) is my metabolism operating at right now? Write this down. ____

If it is less than 80%, then using your fingers to tap gently on the sternum/upper chest, say "I release anything getting in the way of my metabolism" a few times. Continue tapping and then say, "I ask for repair of anything getting in the way of a healthy metabolism" a few times.

Then ask the question: what is my metabolism right now? and see if it has changed. If the number has gone up even a few points, use this exercise each morning to remind your body that it has the capacity to raise your metabolism.

Please note: this is not an exercise to use in the evening. If you find that you have trouble calming down in the evening, you can do a similar exercise saying while tapping the chest: "Now I release my body's stressors and prepare my body for sleep." I also highly recommend using one of Brad Yates' YouTube meridian tapping videos on sleep. (see **Resources** below)

WE WANT TOO MUCH FROM FOOD: CONSOLATION, ENTERTAINMENT, AN EXCUSE TO PROCRASTINATE, A PLACE TO CHOMP ON ANGER, AND A FRIEND WHO REQUIRES NOTHING IN RETURN

Typical Triggers for Emotional Eating

Why do we eat too much? Why do we hold weight? I want to be clear that "eating too much" is just one piece of the puzzle to work with, and may not actually be your issue. Holding weight is another piece of this puzzle. What we're getting at in this section is emotional eating. It's a place to start.

The issue of "emotional eating" covers a lot of subjects, some of which deal with food. We want too much from food sometimes: not just nourishment and pleasure but also consolation, entertainment, an excuse to procrastinate, a place to chomp on our anger, and a friend who requires nothing in return.

As you read through this list of typical triggers for emotional eating, write down the number that says how much you think you are triggered by each one. 0 = no response at all, 10 = very high trigger. After you have done the BSFF™ treatment (notice, test, key word, test) for the sections below, you can come back and pay attention to how your number has changed.

If you are not sure, you can test for each one saying, "This issue of __ is still at a __ (beginning number)" If you get a "no" response, then you can test saying "I am still triggered by this issue." If you get a no, then you're clear.

My 1st date _____   2nd date _____

for testing this asking 0-10:

__   __   Addiction to sugar

__   __   Anger

__   __   Avoid emotions, esp. pain

__   __   Avoiding sexual attraction

__   __   Boredom - Entertainment

__   __   Celebration

__   __   Deprivation/Missing out

__   __   Exhaustion

__   __   Procrastination

__   __   Rebellion

__   __   Reward

__   __   Stress

__   __   Waste*

*(Dr. Peta Stapleton is responsible for most of this list of triggers, used with permission. See **Resources** for more information)

You may notice that "hunger" is not listed in here, but the "positive" trigger of celebration is. Celebrations usually involve food, and there is nothing wrong with that at all. The questions around celebrations center on whether you enjoy the food and the company, or you eat everything in sight because you give yourself permission to overeat "because it's a celebration."

The permission to enjoy is different emotionally than permission to overeat. Perhaps you choose not to go to celebrations, because you know that once you get there, you will not be able to restrain yourself. It is easier to simply not go than to have to deal with the consequences.

All of these issues can be released with

- noticing what the issue is,
- saying it out loud,
- testing for a problem,
- using your key word if necessary,
- testing again, (this can be repeated with the key word as needed) and
- if it does not neutralize, using the Fail-Safe Procedure.

This includes the "addiction to sugar" section. Addiction is a response to internalized pain. (See Gabor Maté in **Resources**.) As a society, we are addicted to sugar. However, we can choose to respond by releasing the emotional pain we've been holding using BSFF™. When we do that, the need to reach for an exterior substance can begin to be released. This is not going to be a one-time procedure, but it can make a serious difference.

As you go through a section, simply note each statement that does not neutralize with your key word without judgment. If you repeat the key word/test a few times and it does not change, work that statement through the Fail-Safe Procedure. Then go back to the statement and see if you have now neutralized it. If not, just mark it and leave it for another day's work. Continue on with the next statement. When you have finished doing that for the whole section, take a deep breath and measure the 0-10 level of your feeling about the issue now.

If you still have discomfort, do The Fail-Safe Procedure for the whole section. Treat any additional issues that you sense you need to treat during this session, and do The Closing Sequence at the end of each treatment session.

Do not be distressed if you cannot clear every part of a section in one session. This is not a sprint, not even a marathon. It's your life. Take it seriously, but also take it easy. Simply do the Closing Sequence, and come back to it. Eventually, things will change. Keep working at it, but give it time.

And if you run into trouble, please do not hesitate to ask for help. This all has the potential for being highly emotional material (as you already know). The BSFF™ process will help neutralize an enormous amount very quickly. At the same time, it is a normal thing for people to want some assistance with specific issues.

The Belief Statements

Take three deep breaths. Now, say the statement behind each dot. Test for whether it is true or not. If not, go on to the next statement. If it tests true, use your key word, and test again. You can do this a few times. If it still tests true, mark it, pop over to the Fail-Safe Procedure, and then come back. You may find it easier to use a stickie, flag, ruler or piece of paper to keep your place when you are doing this work.

Basic Beliefs

- I'm fat and ugly. *Test, key word, test*
- Something's wrong with me. *Test, key word, test*
- I hate myself when I eat. *Test, key word, test*
- I know I'm making myself sick. *Test, key word, test*
- If I don't stop eating, I'm really going to hurt myself. *Test, key word, test*
- I'm so ashamed of the way I eat. *Test, key word, test*
- I'm so ashamed of what I eat. *Test, key word, test*
- Every time I eat, I feel guilty. *Test, key word, test*
- If I don't stop eating, I'm going to die. *Test, key word, test*
- I don't have to worry about being in a relationship. No one would want me looking like this anyway. *Test, key word, test*

- I don't want me looking like this. *Test, key word, test*

- People will know how weak I am because I'm overweight. *Test, key word, test*

- I really need help. *Test, key word, test*

- I don't have time to pay attention to what I'm eating. *Test, key word, test*

- I can easily control my food intake. *Test, key word, test*

- I'm a failure. *Test, key word, test*

- I eat for comfort. *Test, key word, test*

- I can't say no when someone offers me food. *Test, key word, test*

- I can't throw food away. *Test, key word, test*

- This is disgusting. *Test, key word, test*

- I'm disgusting. *Test, key word, test*

- Only lazy people are overweight. *Test, key word, test*

- Food cheating is what I was taught.*Test, key word, test*

- You're only as successful as your appearance.*Test, key word, test*

- Fat is bad.*Test, key word, test*

- Keep count of what you eat, or you'll be fat, ugly and unacceptable.*Test, key word, test*

Remember to breathe. You may want to go get a glass of water, and walk around a little.

Refining Issues

Here is a list of issues that you can use to further refine your work:

- I am holding a lot of stress about my weight. *Test, key word, test*

- I am holding a lot of judgment about my weight. *Test, key word, test*

- I eat to reduce anxiety. *Test, key word, test*

- I eat to reduce worry. *Test, key word, test*

- I eat to reduce fear. *Test, key word, test*

- I eat to reduce sadness. *Test, key word, test*

- I eat to reduce loneliness. *Test, key word, test*

- I eat to reduce depressed feelings. *Test, key word, test*

- I eat to deal with frustration. *Test, key word, test*

- I eat to deal with annoyance. *Test, key word, test*

- I eat to deal with anger. *Test, key word, test*

- I eat to procrastinate. *Test, key word, test*

- I eat to to deal with boredom. *Test, key word, test*

- I eat to reduce feelings of deprivation *Test, key word, test*

- I eat to reduce feelings of restriction.*Test, key word, test*

- I eat to reduce feelings of missing out.*Test, key word, test*

- I eat to deal with exhaustion. *Test, key word, test*

- I eat because after I do something hard I deserve a reward. *Test, key word, test*

- I eat because I cannot stand to waste food. *Test, key word, test*

- I eat because I do not want to deal with sexual attraction. *Test, key word, test*

It is perfectly fine to test, use the key word and test again several times. If it still doesn't neutralize the statement, use the Fail-Safe Procedure. If you have trouble clearing the statement using the Fail-Safe Procedure, simply mark it as something you will want to come back to. You may want to make note of this in your journal. The material below should also be helpful.

While you do this work, you can also ask your subconscious to bring forward any more beliefs that you may be holding that affect your weight. This could be as you are waking from sleep, or when you are doing something besides BSFF™.

Do not be surprised if these beliefs are not directly related to food. *If you accidentally solve all the other problems in your life while working on this one, that's great!* Simply notice, test for whether this is a belief that you are holding, ask for release by using your key word and then testing again. Have your paper ready to write things down - and if nothing comes, it's not a big deal.

You may want to take the list of the Refining Issues statements above and do a short session using that list for a week and see how that works.

Any time using your key word does not neutralize a statement, go through the Fail-Safe Procedure for that statement, and always end with the Closing Sequence, even if it has only been one belief.

Having worked through the above, here are expansions of several typical issues. You can choose a section, or just wade through them in order.

Stress

- I can't lose weight because I'm feeling stressed. *Test, key word, test*

- I'm feeling overwhelmed. *Test, key word, test*

- There's so much pressure in my life. *Test, key word, test*

- There is too much to do. *Test, key word, test*

- No one can help with this. *Test, key word, test*

- I deal with this strain by eating. *Test, key word, test*

- I deal well with tension. *Test, key word, test*

- I'm dealing with this restlessness. *Test, key word, test*

- I eat to calm down. *Test, key word, test*

Avoiding Emotions

- I have to eat if I am feeling anxious. *Test, key word, test*

- I'm feeling nervous about something. *Test, key word, test*

- I'm feeling scared about something. *Test, key word, test*

- I'm not sure what to do about this. *Test, key, test*

- I'm powerless to do anything to resolve/influence this feeling. *Test, key word, test*

- I'm weak. *Test, key word, test*

- What if something happens? *Test, key word, test*

- I feel jittery & restless. *Test, key word, test*

- I can't stop thinking about this. *Test, key word, test*

- This worry is in my head and in my body. *Test, key word, test*

- I have feelings of sadness. *Test, key word, test*

- I feel so sad and I don't know why. *Test, key word, test*

- I feel overwhelmed by this sadness. *Test, key word, test*

- I have feelings of loneliness. *Test, key word, test*

- I feel so alone in the world. *Test, key word, test*

- I feel so alone, despite the people around me. *Test, key word, test*

- I eat because of feelings of depression. *Test, key word, test*
- I eat because of feelings of melancholy. *Test, key word, test*
- I eat because of feelings of misery. *Test, key, test*
- I eat because of feelings of emptiness. *Test, key word, test*
- I eat because I've got no energy. *Test, key word, test*

Remember to breathe. Go get a glass of water, walk around a little.

Food Is My Reward

- I eat because food gives me comfort. *Test, key word, test*
- I eat because I've got no motivation. *Test, key word, test*
- I eat because nothing is enjoyable. *Test, key word, test*
- I only eat when I am hungry. *Test, key word, test*
- I eat because food is my only pleasure right now. *Test, key word, test*
- I eat because nothing can cheer me up. *Test, key word, test*
- I eat because the only reward I have right now is food. *Test, key word, test*

- The only place I get to go right now is the grocery store. *Test, key word, test*

- Right now everything else except food is out of my control. *Test, key word, test*

- When there's a celebration, I get to stuff myself. *Test, key word, test*

- When there's a celebration, it's right to stuff myself. *Test, key word, test*

Frustration, Annoyance, and Angry Feelings

- I know I can reduce this feeling, but I don't want to. *Test, key word, test*

- I'm afraid of addressing these emotions. *Test, key word, test*

- I eat because of these frustrated feelings. *Test, key word, test*

- I eat because of these annoyed feelings. *Test, key word, test*

- I eat because I'm angry that no one else is standing up for me. *Test, key word, test*

- I eat because I'm angry that I have to be the bad guy. *Test, key word, test*

- I eat when someone yells at me. *Test, key word, test*

- I eat because of these angry feelings. *Test, key word, test*

- I eat because of PMS/menopause. *Test, key word, test*

- I eat because dieting makes me angry. *Test, key word, test*

- I eat because low carbs make me angry. *Test, key word, test*

- I eat because I feel "Hangry" *Test, key word, test*

- I eat because I'm angry with myself. *Test, key, test*

- I eat because I feel angry at this body part I don't like. *Test, key word, test*

Boredom and Procrastination

- I don't feel like doing anything. *Test, key word, test*

- I don't have any energy. *Test, key word, test*

- I'm just too tired. *Test, key word, test*

- It is easier to eat than to deal with this emotion. *Test, key word, test*

- Food helps me deal with this feeling. *Test, key word, test*

- I know I can deal with this feeling, but I don't want to. *Test, key word, test*

- I eat because I'm feeling bored. *Test, key word, test*

- I eat because I'm feeling lethargic. *Test, key word, test*

- I eat because I'm feeling flat. *Test, key word, test*

- I eat because I have lack of motivation. *Test, key word, test*

- I eat because of procrastination. *Test, key word, test*

- I eat because everything's too much effort. *Test, key word, test*

- I eat because I need some pleasure in my life and food is it. *Test, key word, test*

Remember to breathe. Go get a glass of water, walk around a little.

Deprivation, Restriction, or Missing Out

- I eat because there is never enough. *Test, key word, test*

- I eat because there never will be enough. *Test, key word, test*

- I eat because there never was enough. *Test, key word, test*

- I eat because of feelings of deprivation. *Test, key word, test*

- I eat because of these restricted feelings. *Test, key word, test*

- I eat because of these feelings of missing out. *Test, key word, test*

- I eat because whenever I have an eating plan I feel restricted. *Test, key word, test*

- I eat because eating healthy foods makes me feel restricted. *Test, key word, test*
- I eat because not being able to eat something makes me feel restricted. *Test, key word, test*
- I eat because whenever I diet I feel deprived and restricted. *Test, key word, test*
- I eat because I know this is not a diet, but it still feels like it. *Test, key word, test*

Eating Too Quickly

- I don't know why but I eat really quickly. *Test, key word, test*
- I am a fast eater. *Test, key word, test*
- I don't think I could ever eat slowly. *Test, key word, test*
- I'm too stressed to eat slowly. *Test, key word, test*
- I'm too tired to eat slowly. *Test, key word, test*
- I don't have the time to eat slowly. *Test, key, test*
- I have to eat quickly so I can _____ . *Test, key word, test*
- Eating it fast is the best way. *Test, key word, test*
- I have real resistance to eating more slowly. *Test, key word, test*
- I was always rushed as a child. *Test, key word, test*
- I had to eat quickly, so I could get enough. *Test, key word, test*

- I had to eat quickly, or I wouldn't get my fair share. *Test, key word, test*

Saying No!

- I have fear of missing out if I say no. *Test, key, test*
- I can't say no because I will feel deprived. *Test, key word, test*
- I can't say no because I feel pressure to conform. *Test, key word, test*
- I can't say no because I have no willpower. *Test, key word, test*
- I can't say no because I have no discipline. *Test, key word, test*
- I can't say no because everyone else will be eating there. *Test, key word, test*
- I can't say no because I have to keep everyone happy. *Test, key word, test*
- I can't say no because I don't want to stand out. *Test, key word, test*
- I can't say no because I don't want to rock the boat. *Test, key word, test*
- I can't say no because I don't want to upset or offend anyone. *Test, key word, test*
- I can't say no because I don't want to deal with their pressure. *Test, key word, test*
- I have to be polite when they offer me food. *Test, key word, test*

- I have to eat the special food they made for me. *Test, key word, test*
- I have to eat their food because that's how they show love. *Test, key word, test*
- I'm not allowed to say no. *Test, key word, test*
- It's OK for me to say no. *Test, key word, test*
- I'll get in trouble if I say no. *Test, key word, test*
- I have to keep eating in a social situation. *Test, key word, test*

Sugar Addiction

- There's not enough sweetness in my life. *Test, key word, test*
- There never has been enough sweetness in my life. *Test, key word, test*
- I love the reward of sugar. *Test, key word, test*
- Sugar is the best reward. *Test, key word, test*
- I can't imagine living without sugar. *Test, key word, test*
- It's too much trouble to cut carbs down. *Test, key word, test*
- I really like sweet things. *Test, key word, test*
- Sweet food makes me happy. *Test, key word, test*
- I don't have time to figure out how to eat less sugar. *Test, key word, test*

- My family won't be happy with me if I don't eat sweet things. *Test, key word, test*
- My family demands that we have sweet things in the house. *Test, key word, test*
- I don't know how to cut carbs. *Test, key word, test*
- I am surprised that sugar counts as an addiction. *Test, key word, test*
- I'm afraid of what will happen if I cut out sugar. *Test, key word, test*

Waste

- I can't throw food away. *Test, key word, test*
- It's against the rules not to finish your food. *Test, key word, test*
- I will be punished if I don't eat what's on my plate. *Test, key word, test*
- It doesn't matter if I served myself or they served me, I have to eat it. *Test, key word, test*
- It's morally wrong to throw away food. *Test, key word, test*
- I would rather eat it than throw it away. *Test, key word, test*

Exhaustion

- I don't get enough sleep. *Test, key word, test*

- It's too hard for me to get good sleep. *Test, key word, test*

- I need to pay attention all the time. *Test, key word, test*

- It's not ok for me to take time out. *Test, key word, test*

- I'm afraid I will never catch up. *Test, key word, test*

- I'm afraid I will never be able to do what I want to. *Test, key word, test*

- I'm afraid I will die without making a difference. *Test, key word, test*

- I'm tired because _____ and therefore I can't _____. *Test, key word, test*

- I just want to run away. *Test, key word, test*

- I can't run away because _____. *Test, key word, test*

- I'm exhausted because I'm not being true to myself. *Test, key word, test*

- I don't know how to be true to myself. *Test, key word, test*

Sexual Attraction

- I can't deal with sexual attraction. *Test, key word, test*

- It's not safe for me to look better. *Test, key word, test*

- It's not safe for me to lose weight in my (body part). *Test, key word, test*
- I'm not allowed to weigh less than my mother/ sister, etc. *Test, key word, test*
- I don't deserve to look any better. *Test, key word, test*
- I don't want to deal with people looking at me. *Test, key word, test*
- It's easier to be fat. *Test, key word, test*

Remember to breathe. Go get a glass of water, walk around a little.

As you have already seen with the Fail-Safe Procedure, you need to pay attention to whether the statement itself is positive or negative.

There are some statements that your conscious mind wants to be true, for example, "I am peaceful with how I look right now ." Your subconscious mind may reject this, in which case the test will show a "no!" answer, and you would use your key word, etc. You are looking for whether it's **clear** or whether the subconscious response is a **problem**. It can be a little tricky.

Stress and Judgment

- There is a downside to my releasing weight. *Test, key word, test*

- There is an upside to my keeping the weight. *Test, key word, test*

- I need to be punished for how my body looks. *Test, key word, test*

- I am guilty. *Test, key word, test*

- I'm ashamed of how I look. *Test, key word, test*

- I'm deeply unhappy with how I look. *Test, key word, test*

- I hate how I feel. *Test, key word, test*

- I hate what I see in the mirror. *Test, key word, test*

- I'm always judging people when I look at their bodies. *Test, key word, test*

- I'm always judging myself when I think about my body. *Test, key word, test*

- It's not ok to take really good care of my body. *Test, key word, test*

- I'm peaceful when I think about my body. *Test, key word, test*

- It's ok for me to be happy with my body. *Test, key word, test*

- I know what my body needs for nourishment. *Test, key word, test*

- I love and approve of myself. *Test, key word, test*

- I am powerful. *Test, key word, test*

- I feel good about myself. *Test, key word, test*
- I am happy with how I look. *Test, key word, test*
- I've always had weight problems. *Test, key word, test*
- I'm deeply frustrated by my weight. *Test, key word, test*
- I'm very stressed about my weight. *Test, key word, test*
- I'm angry at myself for how big I look. *Test, key word, test*
- I feel hopeless about losing weight. *Test, key word, test*
- I don't expect this stuff to help. *Test, key word, test*
- When I allow myself to think about my weight, I panic. *Test, key word, test*
- I was taught to judge my body harshly. *Test, key word, test*
- I can trust my body. *Test, key word, test*
- I don't know who I will be if I am not overweight. *Test, key word, test*
- Guilt and shame are two of my food groups. *Test, key word, test*
- I find healthy ways to nurture myself. *Test, key word, test*
- I am in tune with myself. *Test, key word, test*
- I am kind to my body. *Test, key word, test*

Final Clearing

Go back to what you started with in your journal. In the same way you have tested, used your key word, and tested again, say each statement in your journal out loud, and use the BSFF™ process. Now take each statement and turn it around to the negative of what you wrote down.

For example, the statement "I've always been overweight" might become: "I haven't always been overweight" - and use the BSFF™ process of testing whether the reversed version is clear or a problem in your subconscious.

Suppose you started with "I've always been overweight" as a 10, totally true, and now you test and the answer is 0, not true. Then you test the negative, "I haven't always been overweight" and the answer to that is "true - I haven't always been overweight." When you get a coherent answer to both questions, you know you have really erased this pernicious belief from your subconscious. Keep going with the rest of them. Feel free to repeat, until they seem laughable.

Now, read the following Global Statement:

- I am now treating, in one treatment, all of my fears about my weight and all of the limiting thoughts, beliefs, attitudes, and emotions that would make me keep or take back my fear of what will happen with my weight. *Test, key word, test*

BSFF™ Definitions (especially for practitioners):

A **problem** is a self-limiting and often upsetting personal experience (thought, emotion, or sensation), condition (physical symptom) or behavior (action or inaction) that has subconscious emotional roots (unresolved emotions from the past) combined with a controlling subconscious **belief**, creating a **program**. *Problems are noticed at the conscious level.*

A **program** is caused by a past upsetting emotional life experience, the feelings (emotional roots) and thoughts (belief) about which take up lodging in our subconscious mind and are automatically triggered—like a computer program—as a learned response to current life situations.   *Programs exist at the subconscious level and manifest problems at the conscious level.*

An **issue** in BSFF™ terms is a group of related **problems**. *Issues are noticed at the conscious level.*

A **belief** is something we have decided is true, which is then acted on at the *subconscious* level.

The **subconscious** is the aspect of the mind exists and operates outside of our awareness. It is neither good nor bad, but rather a faithful servant, following our beliefs with action.

A **treatment** in BSFF™ is this: notice, say a statement about the belief or action, test for truth, use the cue or key word to neutralize, and test again.

Fail-Safe Procedure

Treat each problem separately

- I want to be free of this problem. *Test, key word, test*

- I am willing to be free of this problem. *Test, key word, test*

- I am willing to be free of this problem from now on. *Test, key word, test*

- I give myself permission to be free of this problem from now on. *Test, key word, test*

- It's okay for me to be completely free of this problem from now on. *Test, key word, test*

- I deserve to be free of this problem now and from now on. *Test, key word, test*

- It's safe for me to be free of this problem now and from now on. *Test, key word, test*

- I am willing to give up all of the benefits of keeping this problem. *Test, key word, test*

- I am willing to receive all of the positive benefits of being free of this problem. *Test, key word, test*

- I will do everything necessary to ensure that I am free, and remain continually free of this problem from now on. *Test, key word, test*

- There are still one or more problems that will make me keep or take back this problem. *Test, key word, test*

- There is still something in me that will make me keep or take back this problem. *Test, key word, test*

- I am still vulnerable to taking this problem back sometime. *Test, key word, test*

If the Fail-Safe Procedure does not resolve the problem after a few attempts, write the problem down and resolve to return to it later.

The Closing Sequence (long version)

End <u>every</u> session (any time you have used your key word!) with The Closing Sequence (long or short)

1. The Stoppers -

- I am afraid that these treatments won't work for me. *Test, key word, test*

- I am afraid that these treatments won't last. *Test, key word, test*

- I doubt that they will work. *Test, key word, test*

- I doubt that they will last. *Test, key word, test*

- I don't trust myself to do things effectively in these new ways. *Test, key word, test*

- I doubt that I will do things effectively in these new ways. *Test, key word, test*
- I doubt my ability to live out these changes in my life. *Test, key word, test*
- I am vulnerable to taking back one or more of the problems I have treated. *Test, key word, test*

2. I am now treating all my remaining hurt, anger, judgment, criticism, and unforgiveness towards anyone or anything else involved in any of the problems I have treated during this session. *Test, key word, test*

3. I am now treating any leftover trauma or stress still in my being that these problems generated. *Test, key word, test*

4. I am now treating all of my anger, judgment, criticism towards myself for any problem I have treated during this session. *Test, key word, test*

5. I forgive myself for having had any of the problems I have treated during this session. *Test, key word, test*

6. (optional) Thank you Divine One, I give thanks and praise to you for being with me in all of this

Closing Sequence: (the short version)

Please read through the long version a few times before using the short version

1. I forgive everyone and everything - *key word*

2. Now I am treating the Stoppers - *key word*

3. Now I am treating all leftover stress and trauma - *key word*

4. Now I am treating for any anger, judgment or criticism toward myself - *key word*

5. I forgive myself - *key word*

6. (Optional) God/Divine One, I give thanks and praise to you for being with me in all of this

Cracking The Code
Section Two
Crack Physical Weight Codes

TO REALLY CRACK THE CODE, IT'S BOTH/AND, NOT EITHER/OR

As a healer and a nutritionist with a masters in holistic health who has studied weight loss for years, I get rather aggravated with folks who are not holistic.

On the one side there are those who say that the emotional life is where we have to focus. They say that when you clean up your emotional life, you will naturally gravitate towards eating good healthy food, so you don't need to pay much attention there. They basically (and sometimes literally) say, it's not about the food. They're partly right. It's not *only* about the food.

On the other hand, we have the majority of the weight loss folks who want to tell you exactly what is going to help you lose weight with this or that food program (and very often their supplements to help out with that for the low, low price of...).

They usually have something to say about meditation being an important part of it, but not much. We'll get to exercise in a moment. And they're partly right. Crappy food leads to crappy bodies. But . . .

What I say is this: If you're really going to crack the code, it's both/and, not either/or. We must look at the emotional aspects, using BSFF™, meridian tapping, Creating Safety for protection and other body-mind things that work for you. **And** we need to pay attention to which food we eat, and when, and how often.

Eating crappy food (bad fats, highly processed, mostly chemical) will damage your body from the inside out and will keep you from releasing weight. This is not a question or possibility, it's a well-researched fact. At the same time, if we don't deal with the emotional burdens, we can eat all kinds of very "clean" food, and not release weight. It's both/and.

EXERCISE MAKES YOU FEEL BETTER, BUT DOES NOT MAKE YOU RELEASE WEIGHT

Exercise

Let's just get this over with, very quickly. Are you diabetic? Then you MUST be doing some kind of strength training. Period. Why? Because it lowers your blood sugar. It is, in fact, more important than the food.

You can do strength training at home if you don't want to go to the gym (I don't), but doing strength training is **not optional**. Did I say that clearly enough? Did you get that it is strength training I am talking about? Did I mention cardio? I did not. Pay attention, this is your life.

If you are diabetic, find someone who knows something about strength training (the folks at the YMCA do this) and find them yesterday, OK, tomorrow, and start actually doing it immediately. Put it on your calendar for as soon as they're available and you're able to do it (and by "able" I mean *make time for it*).

Can you do strength training at home? Absolutely! In your chair? You bet! Let me give you an example. Find something like a 5 lb bag of flour in your cupboard, or a largish can. Put it in a cloth bag. Now hold it out in front of you, arm straight. Count to 20. Did your arm muscles start to burn?

That burn is what your are looking for. If they didn't burn, keep holding and counting until the muscles complain. Now move your arm out sideways, and do it again, then do this on the other arm. Put the bag on your foot and lift up the foot. Find different ways to make different muscles burn. Squeeze your butt muscles and count.

You get the idea. When it gets easy, move to a heavier weight in your bag. Keep moving from one muscle set to another. Keep counting. You can do this *while watching TV*. No excuses.

There are two more rules for strength training. One, *your release time should equal your squeeze time*. So count while you hold the muscle tight, and count the same time again while you release it.

Rule number two, *don't push the same muscle every day*. Do it no more than every other day. You can do strength training every day, but vary it so that, for example, you do upper body M/W/F and lower body T/Th/Sa. If you push the same muscle every day, you will damage the muscle.

Strength training is a wonderful thing for everyone. If you are close to that diabetic line, go ahead and give yourself a literal break and start doing it. You'll be glad you did.

Now, for everyone (diabetics included), you may have heard "sitting is the new smoking." It's true. Sitting all day is as bad as smoking is for your heart, etc. And, here's the bottom line truth: exercise makes you feel better, and it helps with your *health*, but it does not tend to make you release weight.

You should be doing some kind of movement so that you live a longer and healthier life, and so that you feel better, physically and emotionally. You are **not** doing it to release weight. (See Fung's *The Obesity Code* in **Resources** below for the science on this.)

Those with diabetes are doing strength training, not to release weight, but to control blood sugar. Do I need to say it again? Exercise **does** make you feel better, it **does not** make you release weight. Yes, get out and move, but not because you want to release the weight. Don't expect it to solve the weight problems, and don't give up on it when it doesn't solve the weight problems. That's not what it's *for*.

There are basically three kinds of "exercise" out there. I just talked about strength training, which works on building muscle (don't worry, you're not trying to look like a body builder). There is cardio, which brings up your heart and breathing rates.

And there is yoga and similar modalities, which train you to breathe (more important than we think) and to consciously tense and release the body.

If you're going to do cardio, I'm in favor of high intensity training (HIT), because it takes the least amount of time for the most results. HIT, for beginners, goes like this. Pick an activity that makes you huff and puff, walking down the block, going up the stairs, whatever, and set your timer for 2 minutes.

Do this activity really hard for those two minutes. You should be breathing hard enough that it is not easy to talk. Then stop, usually 3-5 minutes, with your fingers on your carotid artery in your neck, (or look at your device showing your heart rate) waiting for your heart to calm down.

Your breathing will come back before the heart does, but wait for the heart. This recovery time is critical, do not skip it!

In the beginning, waiting for the heart to recover may actually take 5 minutes. This recovery process will get faster. When the heart is calm, do your activity full out again for 2 min. Then stop and do nothing for a few minutes.

After a few days, you may notice that you have to push harder to get to huff and puff. That's the point. Push harder, not longer. You aim for pushing harder for a shorter amount of time, resting, and doing more reps. Your recovery time will shorten, so the total exercise time is still 10-15 min. Nice and efficient. If you want to make it work for you even faster, do this twice a day.

Yoga, Tai Chi, ChiGong, etc., are all wonderful for the body and the mind, if you will do them. Find a teacher you like and a practice you like. Don't be afraid to go poking around to see what might fit your style the best. There are videos galore to look at. Doing a little is better than doing nothing. See if a friend will do it with you.

Movement is important to the body. Think about times when you liked moving, what makes you happy now, and open yourself to finding ways to do that. It doesn't have to be labeled "exercise". Gardening, dancing, forest bathing, what makes you happy?

Remember: Exercise makes you healthier, stronger, and perhaps happier, but it does not make you release weight.

WHEN SHOULD YOU EAT?

Fasting

Let's talk about fasting. Wait a minute, you say, I thought we were going to talk about food. We are — we are going to talk about the **timing** of food, which, it turns out, can be as important as the food we choose to eat. So bear with me here.

When you eat is seriously important. You can now test to ask: I should use some kind of fasting now - Y/N. If the answer is no, please go on to the next section. If it is yes, keep reading here.

You can start your fasting program right now, before you change anything substantial in your food regimen. You can wait until you hit a plateau and then ask the question about fasting again. It may not be time for you, yet. It may not ever be something you need to do. Test!

EACH TIME YOU EAT, THE BODY RELEASES INSULIN

This is not rocket science, but it is good science, and important to understand. Excess insulin causes weight gain. What causes excess insulin? The combination of too much food, especially simple carbs, at the wrong time, eating too many times during the day, and processing foods for too many hours in the day. (See Fung, **Resources**)

Every time you eat, the body releases insulin to carry glucose into the cells to give them energy. A typical

American day looks like this: first thing is a cup of coffee with creamer, then a pastry mid-morning, for lunch there's a sandwich and chips, maybe a fruit, a mid afternoon snack, then a regular dinner of meat and potatoes, and finally popcorn or chips in front of the TV.

That is six hits of insulin. (Go look at how many carbs are in your artificial creamer. If it's not high, look at what the sweetener is. If it's not stevia or a sugar alcohol, you don't want that in your body either.)

Without changing a whole lot, are you willing to drink organic coffee with real heavy cream as your first thing? Right there, you have dropped one of the hits of insulin. Second, plan to eat a fat for one or both of your snacks during the day. That would be a half an avocado, or celery with nut butter, or an ounce or two of real cheese (not cheese crackers), or a fat bomb (see recipe below).

Just by doing that, you have now dropped another two hits of insulin. For some people, just that much is enough to start releasing weight, especially if they have done the emotional release work.

Now look at how important your evening snack is. For one person I've worked with, popcorn is a very special food. I suggested she could add it to the dinner as "dessert" and avoid another insulin hit, just because she would be eating it with other food. Another person realized that she simply didn't have something to do with her hands, so she is now knitting instead of having evening snacks.

A third person realized that he could eat nuts instead of chips, i.e., a fat instead of carbs, a much better choice. Why? Carbs deliver the highest insulin hit when they are alone. Fats deliver almost none. But pay attention to your food labels. Cashews are high in carbs. Slowly chewing raw almonds, one at a time, is much better than handfuls of cashews. Be aware!

What you eat will depend on what food program you choose, but for the moment just let that be. Get used to the shifts suggested in the previous paragraph, and then let's look at the time you eat. How late do you eat, and how early? Most people already fast around 12 hours a day without thinking about it because they are fasting while they sleep.

People often find that when they start using the heavy cream in their morning coffee or tea, they do not need to eat as early as they used to.

Some people find it easier to eat breakfast and lunch, and skip supper. There are several other tricks you can use to lengthen the time of your fast, which is something you may want to do. (Do a Y/N test.)

Here's the simple and important thing to know: your body will release weight more easily when it has longer reliable portions of the day where it doesn't deal with incoming carbs.

So the cream in the coffee is one trick. Knowing that fat does not make the insulin hit much at all is important - it means that eating an avocado does not cut into your fasting time.

Other options are bone broth and greens powder (but look carefully to see if and how they are sweetened). And, of course, the famous fat bombs.

> *Stina's Fat Bomb Recipe: On very low heat, melt 1/2 cup coconut oil until it's clear, then mix in well 1/4 cup natural (no sugar added) peanut butter or other nut butter. Grind up a rounded 1/4 cup of cacao nibs in your coffee grinder (don't worry about washing out the grinder before or after - the coffee leftovers are good in the bombs, and the nibs leftovers are wonderful in the coffee) and add the well-ground nibs to the melted mix along with 1-2 stevia packets. Pour/spoon out into 8-12 silicon muffin cups. Freeze. Eat frozen. (I use Kirkland Peanut Butter.)

Different people will have different issues with all of this fasting business. Personally, I had two issues. It took me 3 days of skipping breakfast, and I was quietly convinced I was going to starve. That was not fun, at all, but by the fourth day, it suddenly had become normal. I loved having that extra time in the morning.

Now it feels weird to eat breakfast. My fast time gradually became a norm of 16 hours each day, sometimes more, sometimes less. Do I ever eat breakfast? Yes.

When my brother came to visit and wanted breakfast, we all sat down and had a lovely breakfast. Do I *normally* eat breakfast now? No, almost never. It's not *the norm* any more.

The second issue for me was snacking. I had no idea I had been snacking as much as I was. I was actually rather shocked at how hard it was when I decided to stop. So, I backed up a step and snacked on fats, bone broth, and greens powder drinks for a good while. Of course, I was doing BSFF™ to release the emotional hits.

I recommend you read "Life in the Fasting Lane" if you want more tips and tricks, and more information generally. It is good science, presented in a very easy to read format. (See **Resources**, below)

Once you have gotten used to your fasting regimen, it's time to decide how this is going to work with your food program, if you have not done that previously. And, if you have hit a plateau, fasting is a good way to bust it, and, I would recommend going back and doing some more BSFF™.

There are two separate goals here. One goal is to progress to no snacking, and just meals. The other goal is for increasing your fasting times, starting with 12 hours, then 14, then 16 and possibly more.

Some people choose certain days every week that they skip two meals a day, which is another way to do it. Again, "Life in the Fasting Lane" will give you more good ideas.

HOW DO YOU NOURISH YOURSELF?

What Should I Eat?

And finally, you're ready to look at food. I want you to hear that **this is not about asking you to eat less food**. Rather, it is making sure that you have enough of the right kinds of food to nourish your body, and enough support to nourish your emotional self. Having gone through the BSFF™ alignment process, and having it available to go through again any time you feel the need, your emotional self should be in pretty good shape.

I have two initial suggestions.

1)**I want you to start off with looking at the fats you eat.** You've no doubt heard about trans-fats, so you know they are bad for you. Anything that says "hydrogenated" is a form of trans-fat. Here are the good fats: coconut oil, olive oil, avocado oil (along with coconut, olives and avocados). Nuts and nut butters, real heavy cream, sour cream and cream cheese for those who can do cow dairy, and real butter and ghee also make the list (If whey is an issue, ghee is your best bet). Bacon and its fat is fine as long as it is processed without nitrates, nitrites, or sugar.

"Vegetable oil" does **not** make the list. If you really want to feel sick, look up how the vegetable oil that comes in big bottles in your regular supermarket is made. If you're up to it, you can start looking at what oils you use at the same time you are learning to put shields up or at any point.

Take the food you are not going to eat any more, and give it to the food bank. It is better than starving. Just don't buy any more of the stuff that does not do your body any good, and that includes anything that says "low fat".

It's fine to give yourself a week, or more, to do this. Get used to using these (perhaps new to you) fats. If you're worried you will gain weight using them, please use BSFF™ to neutralize your fears about this.

2) **Look for "added sugar" on the labels of your food.** Take one shelf at a time, and look at how much added sugar is in the food in your cupboards and refrigerator. We don't need added sugar. In the 1600's, refined sugar was actually called "crack" and now we know that it is as addictive as cocaine, it just does its damage more slowly, over a longer period of time.

ONE PROGRAM IS NOT GOOD
FOR EVERY BODY

What Foods Should I Be Eating?

We are all different, so one program is not going to fit everyone. How can I tell you what you need to do for your food program with any sense of integrity? Here's how — I am going to tell you how to figure this out for yourself.

At this point, I hope that you are fasting at least 12 hours a day, perhaps more, perhaps not, and that you are not snacking on anything that will raise your insulin.

By the way, if it hasn't occurred to you to ask yet, of course you can use BSFF™ on any situation you are not happy with. By using it on a regular basis, you will bring yourself into more and more alignment with the person you want to be, and you will have less stress in your life.

The result is more happiness - a release of all types of weight. Please look in the appendices at the end of the book for ideas on how to do this.

WHAT IS THE TRUTH FOR YOU?

So what's next? When you learned how to do BSFF™, you used muscle, pendulum or Y/N testing. You can use that same testing here. You can make a statement, and test for the truth of that statement for you. So, you can say, "This program would be good for me to do this month" and then test for it, Y/N. If you get a maybe, then it generally means "not yet".

Pay attention to your statement. "This program would be good for me to do this month" is not quite the same as "I should start with this program." This takes a little finesse. Try different statements and see what responses you get. Keep working at it until you feel like you have a strong answer. Sometimes this is better if you try again the next day.

Foods are generally divided into what are called the macros of fats, proteins and carbohydrates. It is the proportion of those that is the first difference you will see in various programs.

The type of protein is another important difference. For some people, animal proteins are important, for others, they are not helpful. If you are not eating a fair amount of animal proteins, remember to increase your intake of Vitamin B12 in methyl cobalamin lozenge form. Again, test for this. Most older Americans are not getting enough B12.

A further note: I propose that there are actually four macros to ask about. The usual three are fat, protein, and carbs, but the fourth is water. If I walk into the kitchen feeling hungry without a particular focus, I start with the sway test asking: I should eat some protein right now. If the answer is "no" then I go on to fat and then carbs, and if I don't get a clear yes on either of those, I will say, I need water right now. After a glass (or two) of water or herbal tea, if I still want some food, I'll test again. If I'm smart, I'll just start with the water question.

There are some "bad" foods, and they are bad for everyone. Some people can tolerate them better than others, but that does not make them good. Take heart; There are not many of these foods, basically refined sugars and highly refined grains (because they turn into sugars too easily) and bad fats.

You also want to get totally off most artificial sweeteners. Stevia is your best choice here. The sugar alcohols (xylitol, malitol, sorbitol and erythritol) are the next best, and they are very helpful as transition foods to help you adjust while you get used to things being less sweet.

Test for which of the sugar alcohols works for you (if any). Personally I do best with erythritol. Usually I mix it with stevia, and flavored liquid stevia is definitely my friend. Stevia packets fit nicely in a wallet for when you go out.

Here's the first trick: your taste buds change entirely every two weeks at the cellular level. What that means is that if you can do something new for two weeks, your taste buds will think this is the new normal. You don't have to go cold turkey with this, just do something slightly new for two weeks.

If you're used to two packets of sweetener in your coffee, first get stevia/erythritol packets, see how they do, then try using 1.5 for a couple of weeks.

After another two weeks, see how it works to use one packet. And pay attention. If you are using real cream in your coffee, do you really need the sweetener? - Maybe, but maybe not!

The second trick is that for most people, your body has a rather low tolerance for all of the sugar alcohols. What this means is that you can eat one brownie made with erythritol or other sugar alcohol without any problems. If you eat three in one sitting, you'll most likely be running to the bathroom with an attack of diarrhea. This is a great incentive to not eat three, don't you think?

So what about coffee? And caffeine in general? As long as you don't have a reaction to caffeine, there's nothing wrong with coffee - as long as it's organic.

Think about spraying pesticides on coffee berries, which are then dried, so now it's really concentrated pesticides: Not good.

Drinking a cup of very good coffee or black tea first thing in the morning with some real cream in it will allow you to lengthen your fasting time. Just go get some organic coffee if you want coffee. If not, a good organic tea works as well and use real cream, not half & half. For those of us who can't tolerate caffeine, a good decaf black tea with cream in it is great, or you may rather have a fat bomb instead!

I drink Prime Tea (see the Resource page) all morning and am quite satisfied. Note: This is not a good tea if you have kidney stones.

WHAT FOOD PROGRAM IS:
BEST FOR ME.
RIGHT NOW?

Please note: The programs I list here are all "good" programs. The correct question is this: Which one is best *for you* to follow *right now*? All of them are going to be very low in added sugar, because refined sugar is basically poison. All of them are going to be using good fats, because bad fats are *absolutely* poison.

Beyond that, there are significant differences, and those differences are important in why you personally should or should not follow a particular regimen. The lovely thing is that now you know you can use your testing to decide which one to start with.

The programs listed here are in no particular order, with my comments on them. You can find plenty of references and books on them. After reading through the list, you want to test, and probably test again for, "This would be the right place for me to start."

Again, *they are not listed in order* - the right one for you to use is dependent on a lot of personal details and preferences. Cycling (no bicycle needed) means you jump full tilt into one of the regimens for a set period of time, usually 2-4 weeks, then back to what you were doing, or on to another one.

All of them are "right" options, the only real question is whether they are right *for you*, right *now*.

> **Prime** - a program of special tea, self-massage and supplements that sets you up for releasing weight with a months-long gentle but serious detox that allows the body to come back into balance, not a

cycling regimen. Can be used with any of the rest of these programs. (See **Resources**)

Keto - high amounts of very good fat, medium protein, very low carb; requires a lot of attention to do it correctly, though you can use aids like Devine's book (see **Resources**); pay attention to total calorie count. You need to have your gallbladder to do true keto. See the note below for issues with gallbladder.

Paleo - high protein, medium fat, medium complex carbs, no dairy or grains or legumes, easier to do than keto, can easily do without gallbladder.

Anti-Inflammatory - a very limited regimen of a couple of proteins, leafy greens, no dairy, no grains, no fruits except lemon and avocado; cleans the system and helps you know what foods you are not tolerating well; after 2-3 weeks, you start introducing certain foods to look for reactions; excellent for cycling. See "Inflammation" and "Allergies & Sensitivities" below.

Mediterranean - a good moderate regimen of healthy fats, proteins and complex carbs, excellent for maintenance, can easily be used for cycling with the other programs.

Raw - 80-100% raw is a "medical" regimen, very good (for some people - so test) for cleaning the system for a month, then move to one of the others, some people can keep to 50-75% raw, excellent for cycling, test for what percentage is best for you long term.

Indigenous - Genetic history can help you know what foods will really nourish you. Now, if you are half or full Inuit, it's unlikely that you will be able to find those traditional foods in the lower 48 states, but it is possible to find substitutes that will nourish you. Read the history of the Pima Indians on both sides of the Mexican-US border to see why this is so important.

Having read through the list and decided, with the help of BSFF™, where you should start, now what? Do some research. I have put some suggestions in the **Resources** section. For the others, look online for guidelines.

With the Prime program, you can go onto The Prime website and take the "gut test", get the book, order the ingredients for the tea and other supplements and then start with Stage 1. The Prime program does not deal with food until Stage 4. You can do the Prime program in conjunction with several of the other food programs.

With the other programs, start by making a list of the foods you will be eating. I would really like you to make two lists, one that is your "eat freely" list, and the second that is the "eat occasionally" list. These lists can go up on the door of your fridge or other logical place, so that when you are hungry, you know what to reach for.

The second thing you will want to do is to continue to clean out your pantry cupboards and refrigerator, so that the things that are easily available are all one or the other of your lists.

It's fine to keep foods that you expect to get back to at some point, or that you think you might want to have if/when you switch to another program. Put them in a box, or in the back of a bottom cupboard. In other words, figure out how to make them difficult instead of easy to get to, for right now. In all cases, you will want to give away most of the refined sugars, refined flours, and all of the non-refrigerated vegetable oils other than coconut, olive and avocado.

In my family, dessert was not optional. When we went to visit my grandmother, one time she said, "there's no dessert, just ice cream and cake." We all laughed, we understood her shorthand for saying that she had not made a specific dessert for this meal. But of course, there was ice cream and cake to be had.

And, at the end of a nice dinner, there was already a lot of good healthy food in our systems, a lot of fiber, protein and fat to mitigate the insulin hit. I didn't realize at the time what a difference that made.

Years later, I was told that I was pre-diabetic. I went through the kitchen looking for everything that had added sugar listed in the ingredients (ketchup!), put everything in boxes, and took them to some friends who did not have enough to eat. I wasn't going to throw food away. I knew it wasn't the best for them either, but it was better than starving. Then I paid lots of attention to what came into the house.

EAT SOMETHING FROM YOUR NEW PROGRAM

Do what makes sense in your situation, but do *something* to start moving in this direction. As I suggested earlier, begin with your fats. And, start eating something from your new program. For most people, starting with a few changes and getting used to them, and then adding a few more, is the better way.

Some people can start a whole new program all at once, but most of us can't. If it takes you a whole month to get fully on board with a particular program, that's just fine. It probably means that you are going to stay with it, because it has become normal. Just start by eating something fun from your new program.

Get your lists up on the fridge or wherever so you can start thinking about what is next.

If you have decided to eat keto, look at where you can incorporate more fats, and get them into your fridge. Make some "fat bombs" and start eating one a day for your treat. Start getting the building blocks for keto into your cupboards. Be very careful of things labeled "keto." It's become a marketing ploy and doesn't mean the food is really keto-friendly. Read the labels.

If you're going paleo, look at where you are going to find the best meats at the best prices, and start eating more of them. If you're going raw, try making some raw rollups for an easy lunch.

You get the idea: Work your way into the new program over a week or two as you get more foods in and out of your kitchen. Then declare that you are ready, get your support lined up, and start.

When my friend decided to do keto, she despaired, looking at the very low amount of carbs she was supposed to eat daily. She could not imagine that it would be possible to get used to eating so few carbs per day. She looked at the list of foods on the fridge again—and then it registered.

There were a lot of foods on the "eat freely" list that she absolutely loved. These were foods that had been forbidden to her since childhood. It was like opening the treasure chest of foods she loved and now could eat.

Giving up the carbs—which she did like—became pretty easy in exchange for the fatty things she loved (gourmet cheese! bacon!). Furthermore, she realized that she was not getting hungry. And then she realized that she was releasing weight.

WE NEED GOOD FATS

Gallbladder Issues

If you have had your gallbladder removed, you may have had a dietician or just some paperwork handed to you that said that you needed to eat low fat from now on. You may have eaten something that was high fat, and had the usual reaction of feeling nauseous and then perhaps had a mad dash to the bathroom. Not eating fat is one way of dealing with that. There's just one problem: We need good fats in our diet.

It's not very difficult if you understand the physiology of what we're working with here. Your gallbladder would spit bile out into the liver when you ate fat, which made it possible for you to eat fat any time you wanted to. However, and here's the secret: the liver also produces bile - but only on schedule.

You get to decide what the schedule for the liver is. The only issue is that once you start eating on schedule, you need to stay on it. So if you normally eat lunch at noon, give or take a half hour, the liver will produce bile at that time every day.

If you don't have your regular lunch and have a big fatty meal at 3:00, you may expect to find yourself back in the bathroom being quite uncomfortable.

There are two ways of handling this, and *you should do both of them*. One is to eat something small at noon, knowing you have this 3:00 dinner, and the other is to avoid eating fat at the 3:00 meal.

If you have eaten at noon, you won't be as hungry at 3:00, and if you avoid the fatty selections, you can avoid the discomfort, and still enjoy being with friends. You do want to eat something at your normal time, to remind the liver that yes, you still want to keep this as the normal time. Just eat lightly, and very low fat, at a "non-normal" time, and you'll be fine.

FIRE IN THE BODY!

Inflammation

Back at the beginning of this book, I asked you to measure your waist. The waist measurement is actually much more important than the weight in terms of overall health. One of my clients released 4 pounds in three weeks, which is good but not an extraordinary amount.

However, in the same amount of time, she lost 9 inches around her waist. Everyone at work assumed she was working out. Surely it was not the food, because she was eating large amounts, a lot more than she had been eating before. The secret? She was eating to reduce inflammation. The waist measurement told the real story.

Another client used the anti-inflammatory program for a couple of months, and then moved to a mostly Mediterranean program. After about six months, I checked in with her. She said, you could have warned me about the shoes! What?

It seems that yes, she had released some weight, and had gone down about three dress sizes because most of her issue was inflammation. So she was very happy about going shopping for new dresses.

What she had not expected was that as everything else released the inflammation, that would also happen to her feet. All of her shoes were now a full size too large.

When you cut yourself, the skin gets all red and inflamed. This is good inflammation. It is the white blood cells rushing in and doing battle on your behalf. Once they win, the skin calms down, and life goes on.

The kind of inflammation that is not healthy is chronic and is at the cellular level. It is literally "fire in the body." There is a lot of evidence out there that cellular inflammation is the cause of cancer, diabetes, heart disease, other chronic diseases and obesity. Please note that obesity is listed as a *result* of inflammation, as is diabetes.

While there are several different reasons why inflammation gets going in the body, there is one resource everyone has to lower it, and that is food choice. Sugars of any sort are inflammatory, as are grains (even whole grains, sorry).

There are some super anti-inflammatory foods: garlic, ginger, onion, turmeric, the hot peppers, and dark leafy greens. You don't have to eat all of these supers, but it is helpful to know which ones will help you the most.

Depending on what issues you are dealing with will depend on how much of an anti-inflammatory diet you want to engage with.

When a friend showed up with cancer, I sat down with her and we went through how to change her diet to a highly anti-inflammatory one. After 6 weeks, she went back to see her oncologist, and he was very surprised and pleased with her numbers. She had been doing her work, and it showed.

If obesity is a result of inflammation, then you can choose to eat an anti-inflammatory diet. The logical result will be the release of weight. If you have also done the emotional work, it will stay off.

PICK ONE THING

Fundamentally, we all should be choosing more anti-inflammatory foods, and choosing less inflammatory foods. Take a piece of paper and draw two lines from top to bottom, dividing the paper in thirds. On one side, the title is "sugars/grains" and on the other side, the title is "anti-inflammatories." The middle neutral category is "fats/proteins." The exception here is if they are bad fats, like margarine or "vegetable oil" because those are highly inflammatory.

Now write down all the foods you normally eat in a day, putting them into the appropriate category. Then pick one thing to change.

And here's the trick: this is a balancing act. If there is something you really want that you know is an inflammatory food, simply make sure you have some of the superfoods in the day to balance out that food. And that takes us to allergies and sensitivities, which also cause inflammation.

Allergies and Sensitivities

Allergies and sensitivities can look the same on the outside, but they are very different on the inside. Someone who has an allergy will respond with a reaction and by creating antibodies every time they are exposed to the offending substance. The person who has a sensitivity will only have a reaction. The reactions may look the same on the outside. Inside the allergic person, however, the antibodies will continue to accumulate until the person may have to carry an Epipen™ in case they get exposed.

There is some evidence that sensitivities and possibly allergies have emotional components that may be treated to lessen the effects of the reactions. In any case, using the anti-inflammatory diet to help figure out what sensitivities you may have is important.

If you think you may have an allergy, you really need to get tested so you know that avoiding the substance is not optional, but a necessity.

Finally, there is good evidence that these foods not only cause inflammation, and therefore cause us to hold weight, but are frequently addictive to us. Look at the foods you crave—you may well be sensitive to them.

There is an easy way to find out: pick a food to check on. Do not eat **any** of this food (read all of your labels carefully) for three days running. The fourth day, eat the suspect food with each meal. So you could strictly avoid wheat for three days. You would not have bread, pasta, etc., but you would also scour the labels and not have anything with "food starch" and make sure the salad dressing and spice mixes were wheat-free.

The fourth day you might have wheat pasta for lunch, a good bagel mid afternoon, and wheat crackers with soup thickened with wheat starch for supper. If you are not sensitive, you will not notice any difference at the end of the fourth day. If you are sensitive, you will notice something.

One of the problems with sensitivities is that what that "something" is can be wildly different from person to person. It also can be different from substance to substance. So, one person recognized that she was having enormous amounts of intestinal gas. When she quit eating gluten, that stopped. Then she noticed that certain foods gave her stomach pain, and realized cow dairy was the culprit. Because the proteins in cow milk are different from those in goat or sheep milk, she can still have the goat and sheep cheeses she loves.

Another person noticed that her face breaks out when she eats cow dairy, and that she has massive brain fog when she eats soy. Cutting out soy is a royal pain in the patoot, but being able to think is more important.

Yet another person was having panic attacks. When she went on the anti-inflammatory diet, she quit having the panic attacks - because she could breathe. She was having a lung reaction to a particular food.

What I want to emphasize here is that the "something different" is not necessarily going to show up as a gut issue, which is where you might expect to find it.

LETTING IT ALL GO

Motility

Motility is all about good poop. This should be very simple. After we eat and get nutrition from the food, we need to let go of what remains from what we ate before. We've been taught that pooping once a day is what we want.

Actually, we should poop about the same number of times that we eat. Here's the incentive: The longer the food stays in the intestines, the more the body keeps, and the more weight stays with you instead of releasing. You want it moving faster - not diarrhea, but faster. So "good" poop means soft but formed, easy to push out, and frequent.

The first thing to do is to look at how much fiber you're eating. Most Americans don't eat enough fiber, and fiber is what makes the food go through easily. Again, this is pretty simple. Go online, look for a list of high fiber foods, and substitute one or two of them. You may be surprised to find, for example, that apples and pears have a lot more fiber than orange juice, or even oranges.

After you've gotten some more fiber in your diet, if you need more help, here are a some ideas. They all work. (So please don't start them all at once, or you'll be *very* sorry.)

Magnesium helps you sleep as well as moving things through. You can get nice-tasting powdered magnesium for a small drink at night. Magnesium in pill form also does the trick. Take as directed. After that, increase as needed.

Flax seed is very good for your body with beneficial oils and hormone support. Here are the secrets about flax seed: When it is whole, it will go right through you and help you poop faster. However, if it is whole, you don't get any of the goodies *other* than motility. So you want to grind it up.

However, once you break its shell, the oil in it goes rancid very quickly. Therefore you do not want to buy ground flax seed. Buy it whole and use a coffee/spice grinder to grind it enough to break the shell, and then put it in the fridge or freezer.

It comes in either brown or gold. The brown tastes a little fishy to some people, but the gold does not. Then you can take a spoonful at a time out of the freezer and put it on your salad, or on top of anything that is cooked. However, take care not to cook the seed. Start with a half teaspoon a day and work up from there.

Psyllium comes ground, and does not have much of a taste. You can add it to a smoothie or, like the flax, just sprinkle it on top of something. Start with a half teaspoon and increase gradually with the flax every few days until you get the desired result on a regular basis (Pun intended).

You can put ground flax and/or psyllium in water and just drink it down. If you do that, make sure that you are ready to drink it when you mix it up, because it will quickly gel into something like egg whites.

Finally, there is a movement you can do that will help move things along. Here's how it works: Sit on the toilet seat, ready to poop. Lean forward as far as you can lean comfortably, allow your hands and arms to relax, and breathe in and out a few times, allowing yourself to relax more with each breath. This gets easier as you practice it, because your body now recognizes: Oh, it's time to relax.

Once you have that initial relaxation, straighten up into an upright sitting position, and pull your shoulders fully up and move back as far as works easily given the back of the toilet. Now lean all the way forward, and back again. Continue this slow rocking back and forth up to ten times. If that is not enough to move things along, try again later.

Why do this exercise? Giulia Enders in Gut (see **Resources**) explains that when we lean forward, or are squatting, we naturally move the poop along through its canal.

Since most Americans do not have access to squat toilets, nor do they generally feel comfortable squatting for any length of time, this is another way to mimic the squatting sensation for the body to realize it is time to move things along.

MINDFUL EATING DOES
MAKE A DIFFERENCE

How Should You Eat?

Here are a few things for you to consider beyond the why and how much and when questions: research has shown that mindful eating makes a difference. When we do not pay attention to what we eat, we actually don't absorb micronutrients, just the macros of fat, protein and carbs. This is pretty wild.

Item A: Researchers took two groups of women, one group ate while watching TV, the other paid attention to what they were eating. The iron intakes were tested, an easy measure of a micro nutrient. The TV watchers did not show the same iron uptake that the mindful eaters had.

Item B: Another set of researchers gave the opposite ethnic food to two groups of women, so the SE Asian women got traditional Scandinavian food, and vice versa. They all ate the food they were given, reluctantly, but again, the micro nutrients did not show up for both groups, because apparently the women did not "register" the food as something that was nutritious. (See numerous PubMed articles on mindfulness and digestion. My conclusion from the research is this: For most of us, mindfulness is not enough of an intervention by itself, but it definitely helps.)

Mindful eating can be a wonderful meditative process where you slowly look at the food, smell it, take a small bite, taste it thoroughly, and finally swallow it.

This is a great thing to try. You will find that you get full on very little food.

However, it is also mindful eating to simply stop for a second, acknowledge that this is food that you have chosen to eat, pay attention to the taste, and then go back to taking care of the two year old. By the time the child is 4, you can start the process of teaching the process of paying attention to food, asking the child about colors and tastes. Obviously, eating in front of the TV is not a good idea.

Finally, we can bless our food, silently or aloud, giving thanks for having food, for having water that is fit to drink, and so on. We can give thanks for the many hands that have brought our food to us. We can give thanks for being able to eat in peace, unlike many in this world. Why should we not stop to bless the food that we take into our bodies? And we can also stop long enough to ask the food to bless us.

SLEEP AFFECTS YOUR WEIGHT

Sleep

I'm not going to go into great detail here. There's a lot of good research out there that shows that sleep definitely has an effect on your weight. So darken your room, use the apps on your computer/tablet/phone to darken/redden screens when it's dark outside (not just when you go to bed), use Brad Yate's tapping videos for sleep (see **Resources**), take naps, do whatever it takes for you to get more sleep.

If that's not enough, do some BSFF™ on what you believe about yourself and sleep: Were you frightened about sleeping as a child, was it not safe for you to sleep, has there been some trauma that happened that is connected with sleep, etc.?

Are you bored when it gets to bedtime so you get involved in a new thing to do and the next thing you know it's the wee hours? Again, notice, pay attention without judgment, write down statements that come to you, and then test, use your key word and see how much you can clear.

This is important enough to spend a bit of time in the therapist's office if you can't shift this on your own, as it affects your entire health. Just make sure they know BSFF™, EFT-Tapping, Matrix Reimprinting (a form of EFT-Tapping) or something similar.

GET READY FOR SABOTAGE

Support

There are different kinds of support. You will know the best kind for you. Get as much as you can.

1. Be ready for people who will sabotage your decision to do things differently than you have before. Understand that they are operating out of their own pain, and that you do not need to make them feel better.

2. Do **not** go into a social situation without some responses at the ready. For example: No thank you, it looks wonderful but I'm taking some medicine that will make me sick if I eat that. Yes, just one bite will make me sick. (what's the medicine?) I'm sorry, I really don't want to talk about it here.

3. When all else fails, look at them with a constricted face, and say, "whoops, gotta find the bathroom!" Because you do, you need to go hide in the bathroom, where you can breathe deeply, calm yourself, and decide what to do next.

4. If the obnoxious person continues to pester you, consider the idea that they have lost the right to your being polite. After three times of politely telling the same person at coffee hour that no, she did not want the cake, my friend said, "Excuse me, but there are a lot of folks here who are diabetic. Why are you pushing so hard? Do you really want them to get sick with this stuff?" The woman blinked, and said, "Oh, I hadn't thought about

that." "Well," my friend said, "you should," and walked off.

5. Set up a buddy, someone that you can exchange texts with, preferably daily, that just affirm that you have done a few minutes of BSFF™ or tapping for the day, or that you have made it through the new food program for the day. It does not need to be any more than this affirmation - and they can be working on whatever their stuff is while you are working on your stuff. This will keep you accountable - and will help them too.

6. If you have someone that you can talk to about how things are going, someone that is also working on food issues, that's wonderful, but if not, at least find someone who will keep you accountable (#5).

7. Professional help can give you ideas on how to implement a particular program. Just make sure that they are in line with what you want to do.

8. If they start talking about "calories in = calories out" you can politely tell them "no thank you." You want someone who has read or at least knows of Dr. Jason Fung's work, and preferably someone who uses BSFF™, EFT or Matrix Reimprinting.

9. If you want to do keto, I would simply ask what they think of keto. If they say it works well for some people, that's fine. If they wrinkle their noses and say something about bacon and sour cream, they probably don't have the knowledge base to help you with it.

Resources

I recommend these resources.

Aeon, The Obesity Era by David Berreby, June 19, 2013 - an extensive article on the overwhelming social and environmental issues promoting obesity, while society blames individuals for their choices

Be Set Free Fast™ www.besetfreefast.com is the official website for BSFF™, books, DVD, (look under the "Intro" section not the store) For training information, video samples, and a quick start tutorial, go to https://www.bsfftraining.org

Chakras, Food, and You, Cyndi Dale & Dana Childs, 2021 - looks at our relationship to food from an entirely different and interesting direction

Eating On the Wild Side, Jo Robinson, 2013 – how to find the most nourishing food in a standard American supermarket - there are some surprises here

Grow A New Body, Alberto Villoldo, 2019 – he's proof of how to grow a new body, this book lays out the whole program if you don't want to spend thousands going to his spa

Gut, Giulia Enders, 2015 – more about how the gut works than you ever thought possible, written for the layperson in a light-hearted style

In the Realm of Hungry Ghosts, Gabor Maté, 2009 – also look him up on YouTube, the best resource for understanding addictions (if you don't think addiction work is part of your issue, just go without any added sugar for a week or two)

Keto After 50, Molly Devine, 2021; Keto Diet, Josh Axe, 2019 - I included these particular keto books because a lot of "keto diet" recommendations are not healthy at all. These are. Devine's book is set up so you don't have to do heavy math. Axe's book gives you more understanding of why and how it works

Life in the Fasting Lane, Jason Fung, Eve Mayer, Megan Ramos, 2020; - takes The Obesity Code, Jason Fung, 2016 - and makes it easy to understand. The Obesity Code gives a clear, stunning and very technical explanation of what makes us fat and what to do about it

Simply Raw, Reversing Diabetes   https://www.filmsforaction.org/watch/simply-raw-reversing-diabetes-in-30-days/ - gives you a great deal of information on going raw and explains how it is possible to reverse diabetes

The Prime, Kulreet Chaudhary, 2016 - The Prime opens up the Ayurvedic framework for health in an easy way; I recommend using her gentle detox (after you have tested for using it, of course)

The Tapping Solution for Weight Loss & Body Confidence, Jessica Ortner, 2014 - very much about our emotional state and how to use tapping for that, not much about food

The Urban Monk, Pedram Shojai, 2016 – walks you through how to live well without having to go live in a monastery

<u>Why We Get Fat</u>, Gary Taubes, 2010 – gives a lot of the history about fat-phobia, the science we need to know, his earlier book is more technical, this one is for the layperson

EFT Resources

- Brad Yates on YouTube has lots of videos on sleep, stress, and other things that get in the way of releasing weight, as well as some directly on the subject. for example: www.youtube.com/watch?v=0b3VadMr7HI and also www.tapwithbrad.com

- Peta Stapleton, https://research.bond.edu.au/en/persons/peta-stapleton - extensive university research on weight loss options that work using EFT tapping

- Craig Weiner and Alina Frank run the EFT Tapping Training Institute www.efttappingtraining.com for great in-person or online trauma-informed training for yourself or to become a certified practitioner.

- Matrix Reimprinting is an advanced form of tapping. You can find practitioners (almost all of whom are online) who have listed their particular areas of expertise as well as training at: https://www.matrixreimprinting.com/

- Carol Look at carollook.com, in her store, you'll see a lot of great abundance products (and for her, abundance is not so much about money or things, it's about what you want out of life - which can include releasing weight.). And scroll down to find her products specifically on weight.

- Nick, Alex and Jessica Ortner's The Tapping Solution - thetappingsolution.com is where you can find both free and subscription tap-along videos for almost anything, including the tapping scripts that are in Jessica's book listed above.

Appendix A - BSFF™ for Life

The regular use of BSFF™ will make you happier, so why not keep using it? The process is the same as you have learned earlier in this book; You only need to change the subject.

First, pick an issue. What one or two things in your life are not going well? Remember that the beginning of BSFF™ is to notice. Step back, as much as you can, and analyze what is going on. Start making notes of what you believe is true about this issue. You can use some of the questions in the journal, like, when did this get started? Who was doing what, and what did you decide was true as a result?

See if you can come up with ten statements - you don't have to even believe they were true. Some of these statements you may have believed as a kid, and now you know better. Write them all down - one for each line.

If you feel overwhelmed, perhaps this is a time to find a BSFF™ practitioner. But if not, you can follow the steps, and watch what happens.

Start by taking your three deep breaths.

Say one of the statements out loud, and then test, using whatever method of testing works easiest for you (muscle testing, pendulum, quick Y/N or 0-10).

If the statement is clear, take a breath and go on to the next one.

If not, say your key word, and test again. You may need to do this step a few times. That's OK. If it doesn't neutralize, pop over and run the problem through the Fail-Safe Procedure. If it still is not settled, mark it, and come back to it later.

When you have gone through your statements and neutralized them, be sure to use the Closing Sequence to close the door on your subconscious.

If you do not finish with the statements you have on your list, but have run out of your time for the day, simply use the Closing Sequence and come back to the work later.

A script for working with grief is included here. In the same way that it is quite normal for issues with a critical parent voice has to do with holding or releasing weight, it is also normal for grief to be part of this process. Change the wording to fit your circumstances.

You may want to set a certain amount of time aside for doing this work each day or week on a regular basis. It also helps to remember that when you are feeling distress at any level, going back and working through any of the statements in the book or in your journal will generally lift your mood. The more you practice, the easier it gets, and the happier you can be!

Appendix B - Grief
Treating Grief: Losing a Loved One to Dementia

Everyone, at some point, experiences the pain of loss. Whether it be the death of a loved one, the loss of a job or the loss of an object with sentimental value, the discomfort can be quite strong. BSFF™ can be used to help heal the pain of loss and allow the grieving person to move on.

For this example, we are going to focus on treating for the pain of losing a loved one to dementia. If you want to focus on another loss, first go through and change the language, then do the process.

Using BSFF™ to eliminate the pain when a loved one leaves us or dies does not mean that the normal caring and grieving process will be short-circuited or eliminated. To do so would not be healthy. However, the grief can be resolved more rapidly and without the usual prolonged emotional pain. BSFF™ can remove whatever might be blocking a person from experiencing and processing the grief in a healthy way. This is all the more important when we are dealing with dementia, or "the long goodbye."

When someone close to you has dementia, you have to deal with the empty space that is created by the loss of who they used to be, the loss of all of the hopes and dreams associated with them, and also who and how they are right now, which can change very quickly. Life without the loved one as they were creates huge grief and fear. It makes it difficult to move forward, and yet we must.

Here are some statements for the issue "I am grieving because my loved one has dementia." Before you start, measure the SUD level of your feelings about your loss of who they were to you. Here again, you can add statements of your choosing to this list. And, of course, instead of saying "my loved one" you can simply use their name. Remember, read each statement slowly and purposefully, feeling its meaning before saying your key word.

It can help to take a deep breath either before or after each statement. Choose the statements that apply to you.

- I am grieving because my loved one has dementia. *Test, key word, test*

- My heart feels so bruised. *Test, key word, test*

- I feel a great sense of loss. *Test, key word, test*

- I don't know what to do without the person they used to be. *Test, key word, test*

- I'm so angry that the person they used to be is gone. *Test, key word, test*

- I'm so sad. *Test, key word, test*

- I am feeling such deep sadness. *Test, key word, test*

- I feel abandoned and alone. *Test, key word, test*

- I'm angry with the doctors for not taking better care of my loved one. *Test, key word, test*

- I'm so angry with God/Higher Power/The Universe for allowing this to happen. *Test, key word, test*

- I feel so betrayed. *Test, key word, test*

- I feel guilty that I'm so angry. *Test, key word, test*

- I'm ashamed that I'm so angry. *Test, key word, test*

- My heart is aching. *Test, key word, test*

- I feel so heartsick. *Test, key word, test*

- I'm heartbroken about it. *Test, key word, test*

- I feel so bereft. *Test, key word, test*

- I've been left so desolate and alone and without what I need. *Test, key word, test*

- I'm so lonely even though they're still here in body. *Test, key word, test*

- I feel cheated. *Test, key word, test*

- I feel guilty that I couldn't do anything to stop this. *Test, key word, test*

- I miss who they were so much. *Test, key word, test*

- I long to talk with who they used to be. *Test, key word, test*

- I give myself permission to let go of this grief. *Test, key word, test*

- I give myself permission to remember who they were with joy. *Test, key word, test*

- It's okay for me to laugh again. *Test, key word, test*

- This empty place in my heart can never be filled. *Test, key word, test*

- I'll feel guilty and ashamed if I let go of this grief. *Test, key word, test*

- I'm willing to let go of this grief and allow myself to embrace life fully. *Test, key word, test*

- I trust that I will be shown how to live my life in this new situation. *Test, key word, test*

- I don't have to be afraid of the future. *Test, key word, test*

- Letting go of this grief does not mean I'll forget the person they used to be. *Test, key word, test*

- I can continue to hold a joyous place in my heart for my loved one. *Test, key word, test*

Here's the Global Statement for this issue:

- I am now treating, in one treatment, all of my painful feelings of loss and grief and all of the limiting thoughts, beliefs, attitudes, and emotions that would ever make me keep or take back these feelings. *Test, key word, test*

Take a deep breath and measure the SUD level of your grief. If you still have discomfort, do The Fail-Safe Procedure. Treat any additional issues that you sense you need to treat during this session, and do The Closing Sequence when you reach the end of your treatment session.

Appendix C - Pendulum
Using A Pendulum
Intro

One can access subconscious information from the body-mind through the use of a pendulum. It has the advantage of not having to do anything consciously per se, rather you let the body speak to you through the movement of the pendulum. This movement comes from the action of the nervous system producing micromovement of your muscles.

It is a matter of holding the pendulum, making the statement, and watching the movement of the pendulum. The pendulum will indicate by its movement whether the statement is true or false as understood by your body-mind, that is, the subconscious.

Choosing a pendulum – neutral and clear

Metal (titanium, steel, brass), clear quartz, and wood tend to be the most neutral and clear energetically, which is what you want.

Once you have chosen a pendulum, it will need clearing of prior energies by placing it on selenite or sea salt. To keep it clear from other energies, it is best to store it separately in a cupboard. You and your pendulum will need training. Once you have trained with your pendulum, do not let others use it—only you.

Stones and crystals have an energetic signature so they will not be the most neutral. At the same time, they may attract you. They will work, just understand that they will not be as neutral as metal or wood. You can test different ones to see how they respond to you.

If you get a lot of movement, like active circling while holding the pendulum and making a statement, that is a good start. Again, other than the metal, wood or clear crystal, remember that there will be the effect of other energies

To begin, a pendulum can be as simple as a metal nut tied onto an 8 inch string.

Training the pendulum

It takes some training with your chosen pendulum to be able to set up clear communication from your body mind. In muscle-testing, a Y/true is strong, a N/false is weak, and a lack of response is neutral. You need to teach your pendulum what is a Yes [positive/strong/true], what is No [negative/weak/false], and what is 'I don't know' [neutral].

Grasp the chain lightly with your thumb and forefinger about 3 inches away from the pendulum, with the palm facing down, with the remaining chain run through the hand for stability. The position of the hand and fingers should be relaxed, typically the thumb will be parallel with the floor. The elbow can rest on a surface for stability, which allows the arm and hand to be most relaxed.

Training involves first choosing the movements, then practicing. It is common for a clockwise movement to be Y/true, and a counterclockwise movement to be N/false. You can also choose forward and backward to be positive and side to side to be negative. Choose your preferred movement.

If you have chosen the clockwise movement, hold the pendulum and say 'pendulum, 'this is a yes, true' multiple times, while you purposely circle the pendulum in a clockwise direction.

Take at least 15 seconds, then do the negative. Say 'pendulum, 'this is a no, false' multiple times, and then you purposely circle the pendulum in a counterclockwise direction. Repeat. If you have chosen the forward/backward movement, do that movement while you tell the pendulum/subconscious what to do in the same manner as described with the circling.

Testing readiness - Polarity

Before initially testing and practicing with your pendulum, check your polarity. (And if you get a new pendulum, you might want to do this again.) If your polarity is reversed, you will get the wrong answer.

Testing for polarity involves holding your hand palm down on the top of your head. The top of our head is positive, and the palm of our hand is negative, so when we place our palm over our head, it is like a magnet with opposite polarities attracting, or being strong – a yes.

To test, place your hand palm down an inch above the top of your head and an inch or two back from what you would think as the center, over the cranial sutures. Now hold your pendulum, starting from a still position and holding your hand still, watching for movement and making no statements as we are testing the interaction of the palm and the top of the head. It should test Y/strong/true because negative and positive attract. If your pendulum swings clockwise, your polarity is correct and you will get correct answers.

Now test the opposite by placing your palm facing up or away from your head – this should test N/false shown by the pendulum circling counterclockwise. If it swings clockwise or if there is no circling, you will need to correct your polarity.

To correct your polarity, put your right hand in the pledge of allegiance position, and where the fingers tips touch, massage deeply while saying three times with feeling, 'I deeply and completely love and accept myself' over about 15+ seconds. You can also cross your wrists and rub both sides at once. Then retest. Once your polarity is correct, you can proceed to using your pendulum.

Using the pendulum

After training the pendulum and then checking for polarity, do an initial test and say 'Pendulum show me a yes', then wait for movement. Your hand should be still, with no conscious movement affecting the action of the pendulum. Then say 'Pendulum show me a no' and wait for the movement.

If you do not get clear answers, there are two likely issues. One is the indication that you need more training. You may want to give yourself some time out, and do the training above again. The other is a reverse of your polarity which you now know how to correct.

A good initial test uses a known answer. Start with holding your hand still so you don't affect the movement of the pendulum, with the pendulum still. To test, say 'my name is ----', your correct name, and wait for an answer.

Always be curious when you wait for your answer. It should move clockwise or forward and back, meaning that is true. Then say an alternate name. 'My name is Bob' or some such, and wait for an answer. It should move counterclockwise or sideways, meaning that is false. Remember you are holding your hand still, being curious, watching, and just letting the pendulum show you an answer based on muscle micromovements. Another simple test might be a statement 'my socks are yellow'. You easily know the answer and can tell if your pendulum indicates an accurate answer.

Hold your pendulum gently with a still hand with support for your elbow such as resting on a table or armchair, make your statement, maintain your attitude of full disinterest and curiosity, and wait. Your hand and arm, thumb and index finger, should be relaxed and hold the pendulum with just enough pressure to be secure.

An answer indicating whether the statement is true or false can come fairly quickly but may take 5 seconds or longer. You may see a level of activity through how quickly it starts moving, and how wide is the circling. If it does not move at all, or vibrates, or moves in a straight line this could mean your body/it doesn't know or the answer is unknown, or it could be a neither yes/true or no/false or dubious, or you are really too interested in the outcome.

This last factor involves intention, the amount of intensity of your interest/investment in the outcome. It is good not to stare at it, or be too interested in the outcome as that definitely can affect the action. Maintain neutrality, and an attitude of both curiosity and disinterest.

An additional reference for further reading is "A Letter to Robin" (https://lettertorobin.files.wordpress.com/2016/06/rbn_10_4_english.pdf).

Appendix D - EFT
What about Meridian Tapping (EFT)?

Meridian tapping is a mind-body anxiety/stress-reducing technique that uses the electrical meridians in the body. It is definitely different than, and works very well with BSFF™, which aligns the subconscious with the conscious mind.

If you do not already know how to do tapping, and want to learn it, I recommend the introduction that Brad Yates gives on YouTube (as well as the rest of his videos, especially the sleep ones). (www.facebook.com/watch/?v=338460073568285) However, you do not need to learn tapping to get all of the benefits from BSFF™.

If you already know tapping, you will recognize that you can use any of the statements in the BSFF™ section for tapping, by simply adding "even though..." to the front of the statement, and "I love and accept myself" to the end of it.

Though they are somewhat related, tapping and BSFF™ do different things. Tapping reduces stress in the body and mind, while BSFF™ brings subconscious belief into alignment with conscious intention. It's helpful to have both of these tools in your toolbox.

One of the very nice things you can use tapping for is to think ahead to the next time you know you will have problems with emotional eating, and tap ahead to release the anxiety. For instance, you are pretty sure you are going to have trouble eating what your body really wants when you go with your friends to the buffet.

If you imagine the scene, and tap as though you are already there, until you don't feel any pull towards the foods that you know you don't want to eat. Then when you get there, you'll be able to do what you really want, which is to satisfy your physical hunger while you enjoy the companionship of your friends.

You can also use tapping when you have run a statement through the Fail-Safe Procedure and it is not resolving. Simply tap a few rounds with the statement, and wait to see if a memory pops up. Tap for that memory, and then go back to the Fail-Safe Procedure and see if it clears. If it doesn't, then get some help to deal with that specific issue, someone who already does EFT, or who does Matrix Reimprinting, which is a type of tapping and trauma release that is very effective.

Another thing you will want to do with EFT Tapping is releasing cravings. Here is the script for doing that:

So - You know the things that usually get you in trouble, imagine that one of them is in front of you. Perhaps it is brownies. Perhaps it is garlic fries. Now make them special, really good. Smell this food. What's your number? If it is under 6, go for something else. Assuming it's more like 8-10, start tapping on the side of the hand:

"Even though I REALLY want this food, I totally love and accept myself" (x3) then tap around with "I

153

really want this!!" Have fun and say the words with emotion.

Take a deep breath and immediately go back to side of hand:

"Even though I really want ALL of this, I totally love and accept myself" (x3), tap around with "I want all of this!!!"

Take another deep breath and jump right back in with:

"Even though I really want all of this RIGHT NOW, I totally love and accept myself" (x3) tapping around with "All of this right now!!!"

Take a deep breath. Take a good look at your imagined food. Do you still want it? Do you still want all of it? What's your number now? Do you just want a small taste?

Here is what is exciting about doing this cravings exercise: If you start doing it, even occasionally, your body will uncouple the food craving from the emotion. In other words, when you get upset, you won't automatically go for what used to be your comfort food.

In fact, the more you tap like this, the less upset you will get, and of course, you can use tapping or BSFF™ to lower any upset that does come along.

Appendix E - BSFF™
Where Did BSFF™ Come From?

This all started with Dr. Roger Callahan, founder and developer of the Callahan Techniques® Thought Field Therapy. He is a clinical psychologist who discovered how to use the connection between emotional response and the acupuncture meridians, and started teaching interested practitioners how to do this.

Both Gary Craig, of EFT Tapping fame, and Dr. Larry Nims, who came up with Be Set Free Fast™, went through the training with Dr. Callahan. Gary Craig is a Stanford engineering graduate. Being an engineer, Craig could see that Callahan's work could be made much simpler. He put together EFT Tapping and is instrumental with some others in the creation of the field of Energy Psychology..

In 1990, Dr. Nims was the first psychologist to be trained by Dr. Callahan. He was one of the very early pioneers in the Energy Psychology genre. He looked at the ramifications of what Callahan was teaching, and went in a very different direction than Craig to create BSFF™. Although he began developing this method in 1990, he first presented his work to the public in 1998 at a seminar sponsored by Craig.

By 1999, Dr. Nims had moved well beyond tapping methods and greatly streamlined BSFF™ treatments— no longer needing tapping on acupuncture meridians at all. Most importantly, he had discovered that he could give a single instruction to the subconscious mind to do the treatment work without hypnosis.

In Dr. Nims' own words: "What BSFF™ does:

- It treats all kinds of distresses and personal limitations—very simply, easily and quickly.

- It works at the deepest level of the psyche to access the subconscious mind using thought energy without any tapping or other physical actions."

BSFF™ Definitions

- A **problem** is a self-limiting and often upsetting personal experience (thought, emotion, or sensation), condition (physical symptom) or behavior (action or inaction) that has subconscious emotional roots (unresolved emotions from the past) combined with a controlling subconscious belief, creating a "program." *Problems are noticed at the conscious level.*

- A **program** is caused by a past upsetting emotional life experience, the feelings (emotional roots) and thoughts (belief) about which take up lodging in our subconscious mind and are automatically triggered –like a computer program-- as a learned response to current life situations. *Programs exist at the subconscious level and manifest problems at the conscious level.*

- An **issue** in BSFF™ is a group of related problems. *Issues are noticed at the conscious level.*

- A **belief** is something we have decided is true, which is then *acted on at the subconscious level.*

- The **subconscious** is the aspect of the mind exists and operates outside of our awareness. It is neither good nor bad, but rather a faithful servant, following our beliefs with action.

- A **treatment** in BSFF™ is this: notice, say a statement about the belief or action, test for truth, use the cue or key word to neutralize, and test again.

Fail-Safe Procedure
Treat each problem separately

- I want to be free of this problem. *Test, key word, test*

- I am willing to be free of this problem. Test, key word, test

- I am willing to be free of this problem from now on. *Test, key word, test*

- I give myself permission to be free of this problem from now on. *Test, key word, test*

- It's okay for me to be completely free of this problem from now on. *Test, key word, test*

- I deserve to be free of this problem now and from now on. *Test, key word, test*

- It's safe for me to be free of this problem now and from now on. *Test, key word, test*
- I am willing to give up all of the benefits of keeping this problem. *Test, key word, test*
- I am willing to receive all of the positive benefits of being free of this problem. *Test, key word, test*
- I will do everything necessary to ensure that I am free, and remain continually free of this problem from now on. *Test, key word, test*
- There are still one or more problems that will make me keep or take back this problem. *Test, key word, test*
- There is still something in me that will make me keep or take back this problem. *Test, key word, test*
- I am still vulnerable to taking this problem back sometime. *Test, key word, test*

If the Fail-Safe Procedure does not resolve the problem after a few attempts, write the problem down and resolve to return to it later.

The Closing Sequence (long version)

End **every** session (any time you have used your cue!) with The Closing Sequence (long or short)

1. The Stoppers -

- I am afraid that these treatments won't work for me. *Test, key word, test*

- I am afraid that these treatments won't last. *Test, key word, test*
- I doubt that they will work. *Test, key word, test*
- I doubt that they will last. *Test, key word, test*
- I don't trust myself to do things effectively in these new ways. *Test, key word, test*
- I doubt that I will do things effectively in these new ways. *Test, key word, test*
- I doubt my ability to live out these changes in my life. *Test, key word, test*
- I am vulnerable to taking back one or more of the problems I have treated. *Test, key word, test*

2. I am now treating all my remaining hurt, anger, judgment, criticism, and unforgiveness towards anyone or anything else involved in any of the problems I have treated during this session. *Test, key word, test*

3. I am now treating any leftover trauma or stress still in my being that these problems generated. *Test, key word, test*

4. I am now treating all of my anger, judgment, criticism towards myself for any problem I have treated during this session. *Test, key word, test*

5. I forgive myself for having had any of the problems I have treated during this session. *Test, key word, test*

6. (optional) Thank you Divine One, I give thanks and praise to you for being with me in all of this

Closing Sequence: (the short version)

Please read through the long version a few times before using the short version

1. Now I am treating the Stoppers - key word

2. Now I am treating all leftover stress and trauma - key word

3. I forgive everyone and everything - key word

4. Now I am treating for any anger, judgment or criticism toward myself - key word

5. I forgive myself - key word

6. (Optional) God/Divine One, I give thanks and praise to you for being with me in all of this

Appendix F - Journal

MY JOURNAL OF RELEASING

WHEN THE WHY IS CLEAR,
THE WAY CAN BECOME CLEAR

This journal is for you. Use it as makes sense to you. I invite you to make notes and date them, and then put something in your calendar that will urge you to come back, consider where you do not have resolution, perhaps make some more notes, and date them. I hope you can easily copy this section and make a separate document, which you can then add to over time. The Fail-Safe and Closing Sequence are at the end of Appendix E for you to print out and use with the BSFF™ statements. You can also find them to download at www.stinasway.com

Begin at the beginning

When you decide to do something, do you do it - or do you find yourself doing something else? What's an example of this?

When you have decided that you no longer are going to do something, do you find yourself doing it again? For example,

Are you calm and stable within yourself?

Do you find yourself pulled this way and that, often irritated and upset, whether you show it on the outside or not?

Do you have a sense of place, knowing who and where you are in the world?

Critical Parent Issues that need more work:

Some Background

(Take three deep breaths - now without judgment see what comes up as your first answer to these questions):

- why do you gain weight?

- why do you gain it back?

- how have you lost weight?

- what was going on the first time you tried to diet?

- what was going on when you first gained weight?

- what was the response of those around you?

- I eat as a response to an emotional overload

- My body has been trained to hold weight

- My body does not know how to release weight

- My body's metabolism has been reduced

- There is a problem in my endocrine system

- It is not safe for me to lose weight

- There is some other issue I need to attend to

Issues!

Rate where you are right now using 0=not an issue for me, 10=serious! on each of these issues. After you have worked through the BSFF™ sections, come back and rate yourself again.

Today's date _____ Next date _____

___	___	Addiction to sugar
___	___	Anger
___	___	Avoid emotions, esp. pain
___	___	Avoiding sexual attraction
___	___	Boredom - Entertainment
___	___	Celebration
___	___	Deprivation/Missing out
___	___	Exhaustion
___	___	Procrastination
___	___	Rebellion
___	___	Reward
___	___	Stress
___	___	Waste

Statements that didn't neutralize easily from:

Basic Beliefs

Refining Issues

Stress

Avoiding Emotions

Food is My Reward

Frustration/Annoyance/Anger

Boredom/Procrastination

Deprivation/Restriction/Missing Out

Eating Too Quickly

Saying No!

Sugar Addiction

Waste

Exhaustion

Sexual Attraction

Stress and Judgment

Support

My primary support buddy is:

My backup support people are:

The places I run into trouble are:

Movement Ideas

Fasting

I'm starting out with my last food of the day at ___ and the first time I normally eat the next day is at ____, so I'm fasting ____ hours. The date today is _____.

Today's date is _____ and I'm normally fasting ___ hours.

Food Program

I'm starting with this program _____ date
_____

How is it going?

Have you paid attention to the issues and used BSFF™
or tapping on them?

Do you need more or less structure?

Check out stinasway.com for more ideas.

1. Current Weight: _____ Date: _____

Waist Measurement: _____

Pants size: _____

A1C or other measures of blood sugar _____
Date:_____

2. Weight: _____ Date: _____

Waist Measurement: _____

Pants size: _____

A1C or other measures of blood sugar _____
Date:_____

3. Weight: _____ Date: _____

Waist Measurement: _____

Pants size: _____

A1C or other measures of blood sugar _____
Date:_____

BSFF™ Flow Chart

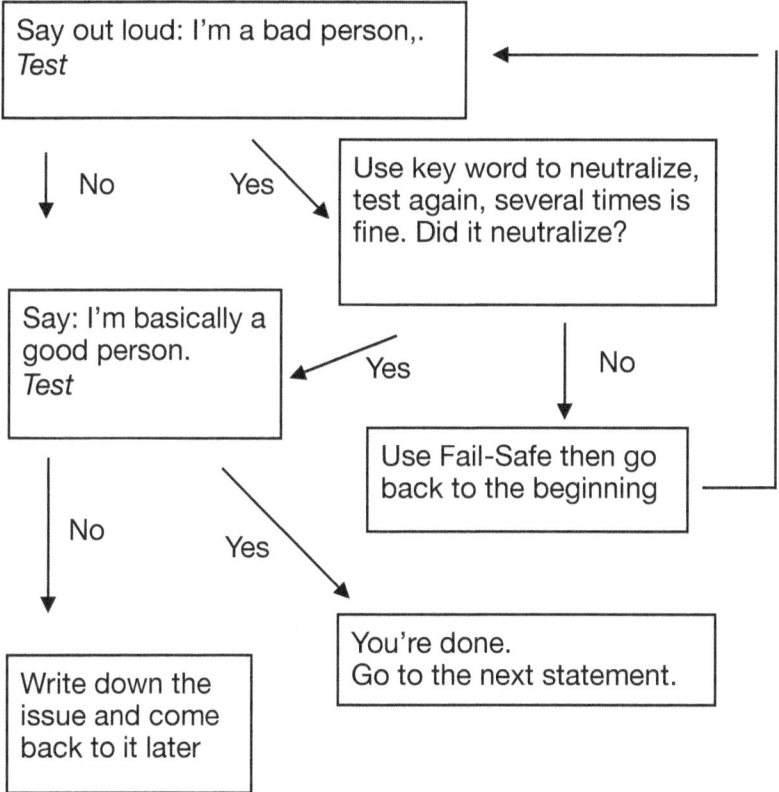

Say out loud: I'm a bad person,.
Test

No / Yes

Use key word to neutralize, test again, several times is fine. Did it neutralize?

Say: I'm basically a good person.
Test

Yes / No

Use Fail-Safe then go back to the beginning

No / Yes

Write down the issue and come back to it later

You're done.
Go to the next statement.

Remember to do the Closing Sequence if you have used your key word!

www.ingramcontent.com/pod-product-compliance
Lightning Source LLC
Chambersburg PA
CBHW022055020426
42335CB00012B/700